Contents

4 Stroke Radiology   32

5 Intravenous Thrombolysis   58

Third Edition

You have just encountered a possible stroke patient. You ask yourself: What should I do first? How do I know it is a stroke? Is it too late to reverse the damage?

This book provides integral assistance in answering these critical questions. All content is arranged in chronological order, covering all considerations in assessing and treating patients in the emergency room, stroke unit, and rehabilitation facilities.

This new edition offers readers the latest information on stroke treatment, and features brand new chapters on stroke radiology, endovascular therapy, the uncommon causes of stroke, cerebral venous thrombosis, stroke prevention, and the transition to outpatient care. The comprehensive set of appendices contains useful reference information, including dosage algorithms, conversion factors, and stroke scales.

M. Carter Denny MD, MPH is an assistant professor of neurology in the stroke program at MedStar Georgetown University Hospital in Washington DC. She completed her two-year vascular neurology fellowship at the University of Texas Health Science Center in Houston, Texas.

Ahmad Riad Ramadan MD is a staff neurologist in the Stroke and Neurocritical Care divisions at Henry Ford Hospital, Detroit, Michigan. He completed a vascular neurology fellowship at the University of Texas Health Science Center in Houston, Texas, as a well as a neurocritical care fellowship at Johns Hopkins Hospital in Baltimore, Maryland.

Sean I. Savitz MD is professor and Director of the Institute for Stroke and Cerebrovascular Disease and holds the Frank M. Yatsu, MD Chair in Neurology at the University of Texas Health Science Center in Houston, Texas. He conducts both basic science and clinical research in stroke, with a focus on developing cell-based therapies to promote stroke recovery.

James C. Grotta MD is Director of the Mobile Stroke Unit Consortium and Director of Stroke Research, Clinical Institute for Research and Innovation, Memorial Hermann–Texas Medical Center, Houston, Texas. He is the editor of the market-leading stroke reference, *Stroke: Pathophysiology, Diagnosis and Management* (6th edition, Elsevier, 2016).

Acute Stroke Care

THIRD EDITION

M. Carter Denny
MedStar Georgetown University Hospital, Washington, DC

Ahmad Riad Ramadan
Henry Ford Hospital, Detroit, MI

Sean I. Savitz
University of Texas Health Science Center, Houston, TX

James C. Grotta
Memorial Hermann Hospital–Texas Medical Center, Houston, TX

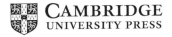

CAMBRIDGE
UNIVERSITY PRESS

CAMBRIDGE
UNIVERSITY PRESS

University Printing House, Cambridge CB2 8BS, United Kingdom

One Liberty Plaza, 20th Floor, New York, NY 10006, USA

477 Williamstown Road, Port Melbourne, VIC 3207, Australia

314–321, 3rd Floor, Plot 3, Splendor Forum, Jasola District Centre,
New Delhi – 110025, India

103 Penang Road, #05–06/07, Visioncrest Commercial, Singapore 238467

Cambridge University Press is part of the University of Cambridge.

It furthers the University's mission by disseminating knowledge in the pursuit of
education, learning, and research at the highest international levels of excellence.

www.cambridge.org
Information on this title: www.cambridge.org/9781108731324
DOI: 10.1017/9781108759823

First edition published 2007
Second edition published 2011
Third edition published 2020
Reprinted 2022

Printed in the United Kingdom by TJ Books Limited, Padstow Cornwall

A catalogue record for this publication is available from the British Library.

Library of Congress Cataloging-in-Publication Data
Names: Carter Denny, M., Ramadan Riad, Ahmad, Savitz, Sean I., Grotta, James C., author.
Preceded by (work): Uchino, Ken. Acute stroke care.
Title: Acute stroke care / M. Carter Denny, Ahmad Riad Ramadan, Sean I. Savitz,
James C. Grotta.
Description: Third edition. | Cambridge, United Kingdom ; New York, NY :
Cambridge University Press, 2020. | Preceded by Acute stroke care : a manual
from the University of Texas-Houston Stroke Team / Ken Uchino, Jennifer
K. Pary, James C. Grotta. 2nd ed. 2011. | Includes bibliographical references and index.
Identifiers: LCCN 2019018727 | ISBN 9781108731324 (alk. paper : paperback)
Subjects: | MESH: Stroke – diagnosis | Stroke – therapy | Handbook
Classification: LCC RC388.5 | NLM WL 39 | DDC 616.8/1–dc23
LC record available at https://lccn.loc.gov/2019018727

ISBN 978-1-108-73132-4 Paperback

15 Stroke Rehabilitation 226

16 Transition to Outpatient Stroke Care 237

Color plate section between pages 142 and 143

Preface to the Third Edition

Stroke is a classical acute medical emergency that needs to be dealt with promptly and effectively to minimize patient morbidity. This book helps answer the critical questions faced by any physician encountering a patient with suspected stroke. It provides practical advice on the care of stroke patients in a range of acute settings. The content is arranged in chronological order, covering the things to consider in assessing and treating the patient in the emergency department, the stroke unit, and then on transfer to a rehabilitation facility. All types of stroke are covered. A comprehensive set of appendices contains useful reference information, including dosing algorithms, medical complications, and stroke scales.

Changes in this third edition include:

- Content moved from appendices to new full chapter:
  - Stroke radiology
- New chapters:
  - Endovascular therapy
  - Less common causes of stroke
  - Cerebral venous sinus thrombosis
  - Transition to outpatient stroke care
- Expanded chapters:
  - Ischemic stroke etiology and secondary prevention – covers information on what a stroke specialist should consider in managing post-acute-stroke patients
  - Subarachnoid hemorrhage – many vascular neurologists will manage these patients
  - Organization of stroke care

Abbreviations

ACA	anterior cerebral artery
ACC	American College of Cardiology
ACE	angiotensin-converting enzyme
ADC	apparent diffusion coefficient
AF	atrial fibrillation
AHA	American Heart Association
AIS	acute ischemic stroke
APA	antiplatelet agent
aPTT	activated partial thromboplastin time
ARB	angiotensin II receptor blocker
ARR	absolute risk reduction
ASA	American Stroke Association
ASCVD	atherosclerotic cardiovascular disease
ASPECTS	Alberta Stroke Programme Early CT Score
AVM	arteriovenous malformation
BAO	basilar artery occlusion
BHF	British Heart Foundation
BHI	breath-holding index
bid	twice a day (*bis in die*)
BP	blood pressure
CAA	cerebral amyloid angiopathy
CAS	carotid artery stenting

CBC	complete blood count
CBF	cerebral blood flow
CBV	cerebral blood volume
CEA	carotid endarterectomy
CI	confidence interval
CN	cranial nerve
CNS	central nervous system
CPP	cerebral perfusion pressure
CRP	C-reactive protein
CS	conscious sedation
CSF	cerebrospinal fluid
CT	computed tomography
CTA	CT angiography
CTP	CT perfusion
CTV	CT venography
CUS	carotid ultrasound
CVST	cerebral venous sinus thrombosis
DAPT	dual antiplatelet therapy
DBP	diastolic blood pressure
DCI	delayed cerebral ischemia
DIC	disseminated intravascular coagulation
DOAC	direct oral anticoagulant
DSA	digital subtraction angiography
DTI	diffusion tensor imaging
DVT	deep venous thrombosis
DWI	diffusion-weighted imaging
ECASS	European Cooperative Acute Stroke Study
ECG	electrocardiogram
ED	emergency department
EEG	electroencephalogram
EIC	early ischemic change
EMA	European Medicines Agency

EMS	emergency medical services
ESR	erythrocyte sedimentation rate
EU	European Union
EVD	external ventricular drain
EVT	endovascular thrombectomy
FDA	Food and Drug Administration (USA)
FEIBA	factor eight inhibitor bypassing agent
FFP	fresh frozen plasma
FLAIR	fluid-attenuated inversion recovery
GA	general anesthesia
GCS	Glasgow Coma Scale
GFR	glomerular filtration rate
GI	gastrointestinal
GRE	gradient echo
GU	genitourinary
HCTZ	hydrochlorothiazide
HDL	high-density lipoprotein
HI	hemorrhagic infarction
HIT	heparin-induced thrombocytopenia
HITS	high-intensity transient signal
HITTS	heparin-induced thrombocytopenia with thrombotic syndrome
HIV	human immunodeficiency virus
HU	Hounsfield unit
IA	intra-arterial
ICA	internal carotid artery
ICH	intracerebral hemorrhage
ICP	intracranial pressure
ICU	intensive care unit
IgG	immunoglobulin G
IgM	immunoglobulin M
IM	intramuscular

INR	international normalized ratio
IV	intravenous
IVH	intraventricular hemorrhage
IVT	intravenous thrombolysis
LACI	lacunar infarction
LDL	low-density lipoprotein
LKW	last known well
LMN	lower motor neuron
LMWH	low-molecular-weight heparin
LOC	level of consciousness
LTAC	long-term acute care
LVO	large-vessel occlusion
MAP	mean arterial pressure
MB	microbubble
MCA	middle cerebral artery
MI	myocardial infarction
MPGR	multiplanar gradient recalled
MRA	magnetic resonance angiogram
MRC	Medical Research Council
MRI	magnetic resonance imaging
mRS	modified Rankin scale
MRSA	methicillin-resistant *Staphylococcus aureus*
MRV	magnetic resonance venography
MSSA	methicillin-sensitive *Staphylococcus aureus*
MSU	mobile stroke unit
MTE	mean time to enhancement
mTICI	modified Thrombolysis in Cerebral Infarction scale
MTT	mean transit time
NCCT	non-contrast CT
NEI	negative enhancement integral
NF-1	neurofibromatosis type 1
NIH	National Institutes of Health

NIHSS	National Institutes of Health Stroke Scale
NINDS	National Institute of Neurological Disorders and Stroke
NNH	number needed to harm
NNT	number needed to treat
NPO	nothing by mouth (*nil per os*)
NSAID	non-steroidal anti-inflammatory drug
NSTEMI	non-ST-elevation myocardial infarction
OOB	out of bed
OR	odds ratio
OT	occupational therapy
PACI	partial anterior circulation infarction
PCA	posterior cerebral artery
PCC	prothrombin complex concentrate
PEG	percutaneous endoscopic gastrostomy
PET	positron-emission tomography
PFO	patent foramen ovale
PH	parenchymal hemorrhage
PO	by mouth (*per os*)
POCI	posterior circulation infarction
PSD	post-stroke depression
PT	physical therapy
PT	prothrombin time
PTT	partial thromboplastin time
PWI	perfusion-weighted imaging
qd	every day (*quaque die*)
RCT	randomized controlled trial
RCVS	reversible cerebral vasoconstriction syndrome
RLS	right-to-left shunt
RRR	relative risk reduction
SAH	subarachnoid hemorrhage
SBP	systolic blood pressure
SC	subcutaneous

SIADH	syndrome of inappropriate antidiuretic hormone secretion
SLE	systemic lupus erythematosus
SLP	speech and language pathologist
SNF	skilled nursing facility
SPECT	single-photon emission computed tomography
SSRI	selective serotonin reuptake inhibitor
ST	speech therapy
STEMI	ST-elevation myocardial infarction
SWI	susceptibility-weighted imaging
TACI	total anterior circulation infarction
TCD	transcranial Doppler ultrasound
TED	thromboembolic deterrent
TEE	transesophageal echocardiogram
TIA	transient ischemic attack
T_{max}	maximum of the tissue residue function
TNK	tenecteplase
tPA	tissue plasminogen activator
tRNA	transfer RNA (ribonucleic acid)
TTE	transthoracic echocardiogram
TTP	time to peak
UFH	unfractionated heparin
UTI	urinary tract infection
VTE	venous thromboembolism
VZV	varicella-zoster virus
WBC	white blood cells
WFNS	World Federation of Neurological Surgeons

Stroke in the Emergency Department

Stroke is the most common neurological emergency, and, because effective treatments are available that must be started within minutes, most acute neurological presentations should be assumed to be a stroke until proven otherwise by history, exam, or radiographic testing. Unfortunately, there is not a quick and easy laboratory or clinical test to determine for sure that the patient lying in front of you is having a stroke, so an accurate history and exam are essential.

■ Is This a Stroke?

DEFINITION

The term "stroke" usually refers either to a cerebral infarction or to a non-traumatic cerebral hemorrhage. Although it will vary depending on the population you are seeing (ethnicity, age, comorbidities), the ratio of infarcts to hemorrhages is about 4 to 1. As will be described in more detail in Chapter 3, cerebral infarcts can be caused by a number of pathological processes, but all end with an occlusion of a cerebral artery or vein. If the arterial occlusion results in a reduction of blood flow insufficient to cause death of tissue (infarction), it is termed "ischemia."

As will be described in more detail in Chapter 12, non-traumatic cerebral hemorrhages are caused by a number of pathological processes which all lead to bleeding into the brain parenchyma and ventricles. Bleeding into the subarachnoid space (Chapter 13) is usually caused by a ruptured aneurysm or vascular malformation. Other types of brain bleeding, for example into the subdural or epidural space, are usually traumatic and are not considered in this book.

PRESENTATION

When taking the history, the most characteristic aspect of a cerebral infarct or hemorrhage is the abrupt onset, so be sure to get the exact flavor of the onset. It is also imperative to determine as precisely as possible the time of onset. The symptoms most often stay the same or improve somewhat over the next few hours, but may worsen in a smooth or stuttering course. Ischemic strokes (but not hemorrhages) may rapidly resolve, but even if they resolve completely, they may recur after minutes to hours.
The second characteristic historical aspect of cerebral infarcts is that the symptoms will usually fit the distribution of a single vascular territory. This is also the most important characteristic of the neurological exam in a patient with an infarct. Therefore, patients with an infarct will present with symptoms and signs in the middle, anterior, or posterior cerebral arteries, a penetrating artery (producing a "lacunar" syndrome), or the vertebral or basilar artery (see below).

Parenchymal hemorrhages also occur in characteristic locations, and usually show the same symptom complex and signs as cerebral infarcts except that early decrease in level of consciousness, nausea and vomiting, headache, and accelerated hypertension are more common with hemorrhages.

Subarachnoid hemorrhages classically present as a bursting, very severe headache ("the worst headache of my life"), and are often accompanied by stiff neck, decreased consciousness, nausea, and vomiting. Focal neurological signs are often absent; if present, they usually signify associated bleeding into the parenchyma.

Signs and symptoms characteristic of the various arterial territories are:

- **Middle cerebral** – contralateral loss of strength and sensation in the face, arm, and to a lesser extent leg. Aphasia if dominant hemisphere, neglect if non-dominant.
- **Anterior cerebral** – contralateral loss of strength and sensation in the leg and to a lesser extent arm.
- **Posterior cerebral** – contralateral visual-field deficit. Possibly confusion and aphasia if dominant hemisphere.
- **Penetrating** (lacunar syndrome) – contralateral weakness or sensory loss (usually not both) in face, arm, and leg. No aphasia, neglect, or visual loss. Possibly ataxia, dysarthria.
- **Vertebral** (or posterior inferior cerebellar) – ataxia, dysarthria, dysphagia, ipsilateral sensory loss on the face, and contralateral sensory loss below the neck.
- **Basilar** – various combinations of limb ataxia, dysarthria, dysphagia, facial and limb weakness and sensory loss (may be bilateral), pupillary asymmetry, disconjugate gaze, visual-field loss, decreased responsiveness.

DIAGNOSIS

There is currently no 100% sensitive and specific test for cerebral infarction in the emergency department, so the diagnosis is usually made on the basis of a characteristic history, exam, presence of comorbidities, and the absence of seizures or other stroke mimics. CT scanning is usually negative in the first 3 hours, or shows only subtle signs that have low interobserver reliability. If available, MRI, or detection of an occluded artery by transcranial Doppler or arteriography (by CT, MRI, or intra-arterial catheterization), can be confirmatory. Parenchymal or subarachnoid hemorrhage, on the other hand, can be reliably detected by emergency CT scanning.

STROKE MIMICS

All of the following may present similarly to a stroke. In all cases, the distinction can be made by an emergent MRI scan, which will show an abnormal diffusion-weighted signal in most stroke cases, but not in mimics.

- **Seizures** – If a seizure has a focal onset in the brain, the patient may be left with weakness, numbness, or speech or vision problems for a period of time (usually less than 24 hours) after the seizure. Unlike the typical cerebral infarct, focal deficits after a seizure are often accompanied by lethargy and have a resolving course, but if the patient has had a seizure accompanying a stroke it is impossible to know for sure how much of the deficit the patient displays is due to each. This is why patients with seizures at onset are usually excluded from clinical trials of new stroke therapies.

- **Migraine** – Patients may have unilateral weakness or numbness, visual changes, or speech disturbances associated with a migraine headache (migraine with aura, previously called "complicated migraine"). Also, patients with migraine with aura are at higher risk for stroke. In trying to make the distinction between complicated migraine and stroke, it is important to remember that because of the high prevalence of both migraine and stroke in the general population, it is dangerous to attribute the patient's deficit to migraine just because the patient has a migraine history. The best rule of thumb is not to make the diagnosis of migraine with aura or migrainous stroke unless the patient has a history of previous migraine events similar to the deficit displayed in the emergency department.

- **Syncope** – This is usually due to hypotension or a cardiac arrhythmia. Stroke rarely presents with syncope alone. Patients with vertebrobasilar insufficiency may have syncope, but there are usually other brainstem or cerebellar findings if syncope is part of the stroke presentation.
- **Hypoglycemia** – Patients with low blood sugar may have symptoms that exactly mimic a stroke. The important thing is to check the blood sugar and, if it is low, correct it. If the symptoms do not resolve with correction of the hypoglycemia, the symptoms are probably from a stroke.
- **Metabolic encephalopathy** – Patients may have confusion, slurred speech, or rarely aphasia with this condition. They usually do not have other prominent focal findings.
- **Drug overdose** – Similar to metabolic encephalopathy.
- **Central nervous system tumor** – The location of the tumor would determine the type of signs and symptoms seen. A tumor, unlike a stroke, usually does not present with sudden focal findings, unless accompanied by a seizure (see above).
- **Herpes simplex encephalitis (HSE)** – This infection tends predominantly to affect the temporal lobes, so patients may have signs of aphasia, hemiparesis, or visual-field cuts. Onset can be rapid, and in its early stages it may mimic a stroke, but fever, CSF pleocytosis, seizures, and decreased level of consciousness are more prominent with HSE.
- **Subdural hematoma** – Depending on the location, this may cause contralateral weakness or numbness that may mimic a stroke. A CT scan can make this diagnosis, but the subdural hematoma, if small, may be subtle.
- **Peripheral compression neuropathy** – This may cause weakness or numbness in a particular peripheral nerve distribution, and it is usually not sudden in onset.
- **Bell's palsy (peripheral seventh nerve palsy)** – The important point here is that the forehead and eye closure are weak on the same side. One can have a stroke involving the pons and produce a peripheral seventh

nerve palsy, but usually there are other signs and symptoms such as weakness, a gaze palsy, or ipsilateral sixth nerve palsy.

- **Benign paroxysmal positional vertigo (BPPV)** – This may cause vertigo, nausea, vomiting, and a sense of imbalance, usually with turning of the head in one direction. This characteristic syndrome is due to labyrinthine dysfunction and not stroke. However, as with syncope, the presence of any brainstem or cerebellar signs should alert one to the possibility of a stroke.
- **Conversion disorder** – Patients may develop neurological signs or symptoms of weakness, numbness, or trouble talking that are manifestations of stress or a psychiatric illness. Always assume that your patient has a true neurological illness first.
- **Stroke recrudescence** – Worsening of pre-existing neurological deficit, usually due to an intercurrent toxic, metabolic, or infectious process (see Chapter 7).

■ What Type of Stroke?

As discussed previously, there are two main types of stroke, ischemic and hemorrhagic. The majority of this book describes the approach to either type of stroke, but there are specific chapters on ischemic stroke (Chapter 3), TIA (Chapter 9), ICH (Chapter 12), and SAH (Chapter 13).

2

What to Do First

The following initial measures apply to all stroke patients. They are necessary to stabilize and assess the patient, and prepare for definitive therapy. All current and, probably, future stroke therapies for both ischemic and hemorrhagic stroke are best implemented as fast as possible, so these things need to be done quickly. This is the general order to do things, but in reality, in order to speed the process, these measures are usually dealt with simultaneously. They are best addressed in the ED, where urgent care pathways for stroke should be established and part of the routine (see Chapter 14).

■ Airway – Breathing – Circulation (ABCs)

- Oxygen saturation and O_2 via nasal cannula. Routine oxygen delivery in acute stroke patients has not been shown to improve outcome. But it is commonly routinely employed, since oxygen desaturation frequently occurs due to pre-existing lung disease, obtundation, acute aspiration, etc.
- Intubation may be necessary if the patient shows arterial oxygen desaturation or cannot "protect" his or her airway from aspirating secretions. However, intubation means that the ability to monitor the neurological exam is lost. The best approach in such patients is to

prepare to intubate immediately, but before doing so, take a moment to be sure the patient does not spontaneously improve or stabilize with good nursing care (suctioning, head position, etc.). Also, if needed, use sedating or paralyzing drugs with a short half-life, to allow for serial neurological exams.

- Consider putting the head of the bed flat. This can significantly help cerebral perfusion. The head of the bed may need to be elevated if airway protection and continued nausea and vomiting are concerns for those with obtundation, nausea, severe dysphagia, or aspiration risk.
- Consider normal saline bolus 250–500 mL if blood pressure is low.
- If the blood pressure is high, antihypertensive treatment is discussed in subsequent chapters (Chapters 3, 5, 6, 7, 8, and 12).
- Be sure to check temperature.

■ What Was the Time of Onset?

- Determining the exact time of onset is critical for establishing eligibility for acute therapies, especially tPA (Chapter 5). It is very important to be a detective. You will usually be told a time by the paramedics or ED triage nurse, but be sure to recheck the information you receive from them. If possible, try to speak personally with first-hand witnesses, nursing-home staff, etc. Often paramedic information is based on an inexact estimate given to paramedics when they arrive on scene, and then gets handed down as fact. You can often help establish the time of onset by finding out the time that the emergency call arrived at the dispatch center, and work backwards with the person who called. Other useful questions are to remind bystanders of their daily routine, TV shows, etc. that might help them accurately establish the time they found the patient or called the emergency services.
- In most cases, the onset is not observed – the patient is found with the deficit. In that case, or in patients who awaken with symptoms, the onset

time is the time the patient was last seen normal. However, if the patient awoke with symptoms, be sure to ask if the patient was up in the middle of the night for any reason (often to go to the bathroom) – as sometimes this puts the patient in the time window for treatment.

■ How Bad Are the Symptoms Now?

- Examine the patient and do the NIH Stroke Scale (NIHSS) (Appendix 7).
- The initial stroke severity is the most important predictor of outcome.

■ Do a Non-Contrast Head CT

- This will immediately rule out hemorrhage (Chapters 4 and 12) as blood is bright on a CT. The initial head CT should not show obvious acute ischemic changes in patients with ischemic infarcts who are eligible for acute interventions, as acute ischemic changes become increasingly apparent between 3 and 24 hours.
- The result will determine the first major branching point in therapeutic decision-making, to be covered in the subsequent chapters.
- Obtaining the CT is often the major impediment in preparing for thrombolytic therapy, so efforts should be made to shorten "door to CT" time, which should be below 30 minutes. For instance, we allow the triage nurse to order the CT scan if a stroke is suspected, and stroke patients will get preference over any other patient for CT access. Another problem is prompt reading of CT scans, especially in small hospitals in rural communities. Make sure to notify the reading radiologist that this patient is a possible tPA candidate.
- In some select centers, emergency MRI can be done very quickly and substitute for CT, but this is the exception. In general, MRI is deferred until after the first decision is made whether to treat with tPA.

■ If the CT Shows No Blood, Try to Get the Artery Open

- Intravenous tPA and endovascular thrombectomy (EVT) are the only FDA-approved treatments for ischemic stroke. They are highly effective but require several preparatory steps, so you should immediately begin to determine if the patient is eligible for these therapies and prepare for their administration. The tPA protocol is described in Chapter 5, and EVT in Chapter 6.

■ Recommended Diagnostic Evaluation

- Current American Stroke Association (ASA) guidelines are unclear about the required diagnostic studies for immediate use in a patient with suspected acute ischemic stroke.[1] We recommend that the following should be ordered in the ED, but you should not delay tPA treatment waiting for results once the patient meets established criteria (Chapter 5).

ALL PATIENTS

- non-contrast brain CT or brain MRI
- blood glucose
- serum electrolytes/renal/liver function tests[*]
- ECG and cardiac monitoring[*]
- complete blood count, including platelet count[†]

[*] It is not necessary to know the results of these tests before giving tPA.

[†] Thrombolytic therapy should not be delayed while awaiting the results unless there is clinical suspicion of a bleeding abnormality or thrombocytopenia, the patient has received heparin or warfarin, or use of anticoagulants is not known but suspected based on history or clinical presentation.

- prothrombin time/INR[†]
- activated partial thromboplastin time[†]

MOST PATIENTS

- vascular imaging (CTA, MRA, or DSA)
- echocardiography

SELECTED PATIENTS

- markers of cardiac ischemia
- toxicology screen
- blood alcohol level
- pregnancy test
- arterial blood gas tests (if hypoxia is suspected)
- chest radiography (if lung disease is suspected)
- lumbar puncture (if subarachnoid hemorrhage is suspected and CT is negative for blood)
- electroencephalogram (if seizures are suspected)

References

1 Powers WJ, Rabinstein AA, Ackerson T, *et al.*; American Heart Association Stroke Council. 2018 guidelines for the early management of patients with acute ischemic stroke: a guideline for healthcare professionals from the American Heart Association/ American Stroke Association. *Stroke* 2018; 49: e46–e110.

3

Ischemic Stroke

This chapter discusses the four main components of acute ischemic stroke care. The sections on prevention of complications, and recovery and rehabilitation, are applicable to both ischemic and hemorrhagic stroke patients.

■ Definition

An ischemic stroke is death of brain tissue due to interruption of blood flow to a region of the brain, caused by occlusion of a cerebral or cervical artery or, less likely, a cerebral vein.

■ Etiology

The etiology of the ischemic stroke is important, to help determine the best treatment to prevent another stroke. However, regardless of etiology, initial therapy is for the most part the same, and so initially the most important thing is to implement the acute measures described in this chapter.

■ Diagnosis

The first important task is to differentiate between ischemic and hemorrhagic stroke, which can be done with a head CT. Detailed brain and vascular imaging are critically important, but should not delay assessment for tPA candidacy. There are things that can mimic stroke (see Chapter 1), and a focused history should quickly exclude these. Unless the presentation is atypical or a stroke mimic is suggested, one should assume it is a stroke and proceed with the determination of whether or not the patient is a candidate for acute therapy. A detailed diagnostic evaluation should be deferred (Chapter 2).

■ The Four Components of Ischemic Stroke Care

There are four components to caring for people with acute ischemic stroke. At every point, you should be thinking about the four issues:

1. Acute therapy and optimization of neurological status
2. Prevention of neurological deterioration or medical complications
3. Etiological work-up for secondary prevention
4. Recovery and rehabilitation

This chapter discusses the four components in brief, and then there are longer discussions of each in subsequent chapters:

- Reperfusion – tPA and EVT (Chapters 5 and 6)
- Neurological deterioration (Chapter 7)
- Etiology and secondary prevention (Chapter 8)
- Rehabilitation and recovery (Chapters 15 and 16)

See also Appendix 3, *Medical Complications*.

■ Acute Therapy and Optimization of Neurological Status

The main goal of therapy is to get the artery open and re-establish blood flow. You should always ask yourself if you are doing everything possible to optimize blood flow to regions of cerebral ischemia.

INTRAVENOUS RECOMBINANT TISSUE PLASMINOGEN ACTIVATOR (tPA) AND ENDOVASCULAR THROMBECTOMY (EVT)

In this book, we will refer to recombinant tissue plasminogen activator as tPA, because that is what it is usually called in the busy emergency department. However, the reader should be aware that this drug is also referred to as rt-PA, t-PA, TPA, alteplase (generic name), or Activase or Actilyse (trade names).

- Details of the tPA protocol can be found in Chapter 5.
- Intravenous tPA within 3 hours of stroke onset is approved by the regulatory bodies (FDA in the USA, EMA in the EU) for acute ischemic stroke in the USA, European Union, and many other countries.
- Intravenous tPA between 3 and 4.5 hours after stroke onset was effective in a randomized clinical trial and is incorporated in the guideline recommendations by the American Stroke Association (class I recommendation, level of evidence B)[1] and the European Stroke Organisation (class I recommendation, level of evidence A).[2]
- EVT is a highly effective FDA-approved intervention for patients with large-vessel occlusion (LVO), namely the distal internal carotid or proximal middle cerebral arteries. EVT is covered in detail in Chapter 6.

CONCURRENT DIAGNOSTIC TESTING

Determination of stroke etiology is usually deferred until after starting tPA therapy. However, while considering or instituting tPA, concomitant information about vascular and tissue status is important for deciding about the need for EVT. The following diagnostic tests may be helpful in determining the stroke mechanism; however, the need to do acute studies depends on a balance of availability of therapy, time requirement, clinical suspicion, and cost. See Chapter 4 for detailed descriptions of the following radiological tests:

- Head CT should already have been done, as it is one of the vital first steps in the management of the stroke patient and helps to exclude hemorrhage.

- CT angiography (CTA) can quickly provide a snapshot of the entire cerebral arterial anatomy, and can diagnose intracranial and extracranial stenoses, aneurysms, or dissections. It is the most frequently employed test for detecting LVO and EVT eligibility. In some centers, it may be necessary to know the patient's creatinine prior to the administration of IV contrast, though this is no longer required in current guidelines. It is also necessary to exclude a contrast allergy.

- CT perfusion (CTP) gives a spatial representation of cerebral perfusion. Software packages include measurement of time delay from bolus to arrival of dye into the brain and the amount of dye in the affected region compared to the opposite side. These parameters can be thresholded to reflect ischemic tissue at risk and tissue where flow is so low that irreversible damage is likely. However, CTP requires more contrast, more radiation, more patient cooperation, and a larger-bore peripheral IV access.

- MR angiography (MRA) of the neck and circle of Willis provides the same information as CTA without risk of contrast. However, patients must be cooperative to hold still for several minutes, and those with a pacemaker and some with aneurysm clips or stents may not be eligible for MRI scanning.

- Transcranial Doppler ultrasound (TCD) can be performed to detect occlusion, recanalization, and reocclusion of the large intracranial arteries in real time and can be brought to the patient's bedside in the emergency department (Appendix 2). However, this test is usually not available in the ED, and it is not as accurate as CTA or MRA (see below) for establishing the presence and location of LVO.

- MR imaging (MRI) of the brain can provide substantial information on stroke localization, age, bleeding, and tissue status. However, the same caveats apply as with MRA.

MAINTENANCE OF CEREBRAL PERFUSION

To maximize brain perfusion through stenoses and collateral vessels, we maintain euvolemia and support blood pressure.

Do not treat hypertension acutely unless:

1. the patient is otherwise a tPA candidate

or

2. the patient has acute hypertensive end organ damage (congestive heart failure, myocardial infarction, hypertensive encephalopathy, dissecting aortic aneurysm, etc.)

or

3. systolic or diastolic pressures are above 220 or 120 mmHg, respectively.

If you are going to treat hypertension, consider using a short-acting IV agent that will wear off quickly or be turned off in case BP drops too much, such as:

- labetalol (Trandate, Normodyne) 10–20 mg IV
- nicardipine (Cardene) 5 mg/h IV infusion as initial dose; titrate to desired effect by increasing 2.5 mg/h every 5 minutes to maximum of 15 mg/h

Goal: blood pressure reduction by 10–15%.

or

- treat hypertension slowly with oral or enteral rather than intravenous antihypertensives.

Don't forget to write BP goals for the nurses to follow that include both lower and upper limits for SBP and DBP.

In the absence of controlled prospective data, there is some consensus but still significant uncertainty about what levels of blood pressure to treat,

Table 3.1 Management of blood pressure before and after intravenous tPA or other acute reperfusion intervention

1. Before tPA bolus and during tPA infusion

Blood-pressure level: systolic > 185 mmHg or diastolic > 110 mmHg

- Labetalol 10–20 mg IV over 1–2 minutes, may repeat × 1

  or

- Nicardipine infusion, 5 mg/h, titrate up by 2.5 mg/h at 5- to 15-minute intervals, maximum dose 15 mg/h; when desired blood pressure attained, reduce to 3 mg/h

  or

- Clevidipine infusion, 1–2 mg/h, titrate up by doubling the dose every 2–5 minutes until goal BP is reached; maximum dose 21 mg/h

If blood pressure does not decline and remains > 185/110 mmHg, do not administer tPA

2. After tPA infusion

Monitor blood pressure every 15 minutes during treatment and then for another 2 hours, then every 30 minutes for 6 hours, and then every hour for 16 hours

Blood-pressure level: systolic > 180 mmHg or diastolic > 105 mmHg

- Nicardipine infusion, 5 mg/h, titrate up by 2.5 mg/h at 5- to 15-minute intervals, maximum dose 15 mg/h; when desired blood pressure attained, reduce to 3 mg/h

  or

- Labetalol 10 mg IV followed by an infusion at 2–8 mg/min

  or

- Clevidipine infusion, 1–2 mg/h, titrate up by doubling the dose every 2–5 minutes until goal BP is reached; maximum dose 21 mg/h

Source: Stroke 2018; 49: e46–e110. © 2018 American Heart Association, Inc. Reprinted with permission.

how fast to lower the pressure, and what drugs to use (see Chapter 8). In tPA candidates, we follow the guidelines in Table 3.1; we use nicardipine most commonly in the ED and during the first 24 hours to titrate blood pressure smoothly to desired levels.

Other options for maintenance of cerebral perfusion include:

- Normal saline for IV fluids – to maintain euvolemia and because it is isotonic and will not cause fluid shifts:
  - normal saline 500 mL bolus over 20–30 minutes
- Adjust head position. A recent study suggested no benefit of routine head lowering, but included mainly minor strokes.[3] In patients with LVO or who are fluctuating, laying the head of the bed flat may be beneficial.

ANTIPLATELET AND ANTICOAGULANT THERAPY AS AN ACUTE TREATMENT FOR ISCHEMIC STROKE

Both antiplatelet and anticoagulant therapy are often considered in the acute therapy of ischemic stroke, and one or both may be appropriate, but randomized trials have shown that anticoagulants should not be routinely employed acutely. Trials have shown that antiplatelets have only a modest benefit, and no studies have yet shown the benefit of urgent antiplatelet treatment.

Acute Antiplatelet Therapy

Aspirin for acute stroke has been shown to have only a marginal effect on improving stroke outcome when studied in thousands of patients.

Antiplatelet treatment is mainly intended for secondary stroke prevention and is covered in Chapter 8. Antiplatelets should be started within the first 24 hours after stroke onset unless there is active bleeding or other contraindication, since the risk of recurrent stroke is the highest in the first 2 weeks after the index event. Current guidelines recommend aspirin 81–325 mg. However, based on recent randomized trials, the trend is to treat more patients with non-cardioembolic strokes with the combination of aspirin 81 mg + clopidogrel (300–600 mg loading dose followed by 75 mg) for anywhere from 3 weeks to 3 months during the period of highest recurrent stroke risk, and then a single antiplatelet after that. The rationale and duration of antiplatelet therapy according to stroke etiology is discussed in Chapter 8.

Patients who have increased bleeding risk should only receive monotherapy. Long-term dual antiplatelet therapy is generally not recommended because of the increased risk of bleeding.

Acute Anticoagulant Therapy

Anticoagulation for acute ischemic stroke has never been shown to be effective. Even among those with atrial fibrillation, the stroke recurrence rate is only ~5–8% in the first 14 days, which is not reduced by early acute anticoagulation.

Anticoagulation is mostly used for long-term secondary prevention in patients with atrial fibrillation and cardioembolic stroke at this point. Without convincing supporting data, some clinicians advocate acute anticoagulation with heparin in certain cases. These include patients with a cardioembolic condition at high risk for recurrence (thrombus on valves, metallic prosthetic valves, or mural thrombus), documented large-artery (ICA, MCA, or basilar artery) occlusive clot at risk for distal embolism, arterial dissection, or venous thrombosis. Such patients may be started on heparin acutely and transitioned to warfarin (Coumadin) or a direct thrombin inhibitor (dabigatran) or factor Xa inhibitor (rivaroxaban, apixaban, or edoxaban). If ordering heparin, use a weight-adjusted algorithm with no bolus. Enoxaparin (Lovenox) at 1 mg/kg subcutaneously every 12 hours may be used in place of heparin. The direct thrombin or Xa inhibitors avoid the need to use adjusted heparin or enoxaparin to "bridge" until the INR reaches the goal level. However, because of the risk of promoting hemorrhagic conversion, we generally recommend against heparin "bridging" unless the patient has one of the conditions listed above that increase the risk of re-embolization.[4]

How Long Should You Wait Before Starting Anticoagulation?

There are no clear data on this topic. There is concern that the risk of hemorrhagic conversion is increased with anticoagulation, particularly in patients with large strokes. Hemorrhagic transformation is frequent in the

evolution of large infarcts, especially those that have been reperfused
either by spontaneous recanalization or with thrombolytics. One should
be particularly careful about early anticoagulation in these patients. We
generally wait 2–14 days before starting anticoagulation, the specific
duration depending on the urgency of the indication versus the risks. You
must carefully weigh the risks and benefits on a case-by-case basis, and
never start anticoagulants without obtaining brain imaging first, to
exclude ongoing hemorrhagic evolution or brain swelling.

HYPERGLYCEMIA

Hyperglycemia is known to worsen stroke outcome. The mechanism by which
and the level at which hyperglycemia worsens stroke are not known. However,
there are data that show even modest hyperglycemia (glucose > 150 mg/dL)
enlarges eventual stroke size and increases the risk of brain hemorrhage. The
American Stroke Association recommends therapy for persistent
hyperglycemia > 140 mg/dL (class II recommendation),[1] and European
guidelines recommend it at > 180 mg/dL (class IV).[2] Hyperglycemia may be
particularly important in patients treated with reperfusion therapies. A recent
study showed that aggressive glucose correction to 80–130 mg/dL is not
beneficial.[5] The rapidity of treatment (insulin infusion or not), the goal glucose
level, and the duration remain uncertain.

HYPERTHERMIA

While studies of induced hypothermia have shown that complications,
especially pneumonia, obviate any benefit, it is clear that hyperthermia is
associated with worse outcome. Experimentally, increasing the body
temperature of animals increases metabolic demand and infarct size.
Therefore, treat hyperthermia aggressively with acetaminophen (Tylenol)
and cooling blankets if necessary.

■ Etiological Work-up for Secondary Prevention

See also Chapter 8, which covers in more detail the evaluation of stroke patients and how to choose secondary prevention strategies in relation to the results of the diagnostic tests.

With brain imaging and vascular evaluation we try to find a *specific etiology* such as cardioembolic source, arterial stenosis, etc. (Figure 3.1).

At the same time, we look for reversible *risk factors* for recurrent stroke, such as hypertension, diabetes, hypercholesterolemia, and smoking/substance abuse that will need to be addressed.

There are several different ways to classify strokes (based on severity, location, size, etc.), but for planning a secondary stroke prevention strategy we find the following TOAST classification most useful, since it is based on the stroke mechanism:[7]

- **Large-artery atherosclerosis** – intracranial, extracranial (carotid, vertebral, aortic arch)
- **Cardioembolic** – atrial fibrillation, segmental wall akinesis, paradoxical embolus, etc.
- **Small vessel** – lacunar infarction
- **Other** – unusual causes (dissection, venous thrombosis, drugs, etc.)
- **Unknown** – cryptogenic. Within this category there is a subgroup recently defined "embolic stroke of unknown source" (ESUS).

SCREENING FOR ARTERIAL STENOSIS/OBSTRUCTION

Recent guidelines have questioned the cost-effectiveness of routine vascular imaging in stroke patients, but we feel that it is essential to understand the etiology of the stroke in order to effectively treat it and design secondary stroke prevention. Therefore, we recommend some

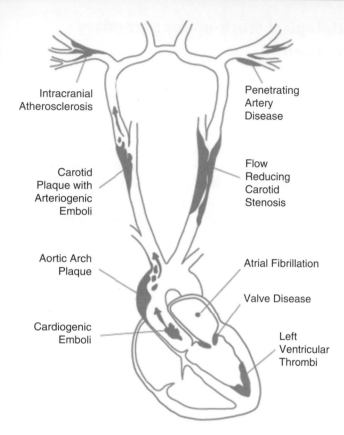

Figure 3.1 Mechanisms of ischemic stroke. (A black and white version of this figure will appear in some formats. For the color version, please refer to the plate section.)
Source: Albers GW, Amarenco P, Easton JD, Sacco RL, Teal P. Antithrombotic and thrombolytic therapy for ischemic stroke: the Seventh ACCP Conference on Antithrombotic and Thrombolytic Therapy. *Chest* 2004; 126 (3 suppl): 483S–512S.[6] Reproduced with permission.

form of vascular imaging in most ischemic stroke patients. Imaging will be discussed in more detail in Chapter 4.

CARDIAC EVALUATION

Similarly, recent guidelines have questioned the cost-effectiveness of routine cardiac evaluation in stroke patients. However, at least an electrocardiogram (ECG) and initial cardiac monitoring should be carried out in most ischemic stroke patients, for several reasons. First is the frequent coassociation of cardiovascular disease in patients with cerebrovascular disease. Second is that the majority of severe strokes are on an embolic basis, and discovering a cardiac source of embolus will trigger very effective preventive measures that will reduce the risk of subsequent disability. An ECG done in close proximity to stroke onset may detect atrial fibrillation and also rule out silent myocardial infarction or ischemia which may occur as a consequence of the stroke. More extended cardiac monitoring with either an external or an implanted monitoring device should be considered if atrial fibrillation or other important arrhythmia is suspected on the basis of either the ECG or clinical/imaging stroke profile.

An echocardiogram is helpful in looking for a cardioembolic source and right-to-left shunts in patients with an embolic stroke profile. A transthoracic echocardiogram (TTE) can show wall motion abnormalities (anterior wall akinesis carries high embolic risk), low left ventricular ejection fraction (< 20–30% generally agreed upon as a cutoff), valvular abnormalities, and a patent foramen ovale (PFO). A transesophageal echocardiogram (TEE) can show the atria better. Left atrial appendage clot, size of PFO, PFO associated with atrial septal aneurysm, aortic arch atheroma, and spontaneous echo contrast are some of the findings associated with increased risk for ischemic stroke. TCD with bubble contrast is as sensitive as TEE for detection of right-to-left shunt.

RECURRENT STROKE RISK FACTOR SCREENING

- Monitor blood pressure.
- Obtain fasting lipid panel.

- Screen for diabetes.
- Smoking cessation counseling, if applicable.

■ Prevention of Neurological Deterioration or Medical Complications

Neurological deterioration and medical complications are covered in more detail in Chapter 7 and Appendix 3.

The following measures should be instituted in all stroke patients:

- Deep venous thrombosis (DVT) prophylaxis (pharmacologic, devices, patient mobilization).
- Aspiration precautions (swallowing assessment and nursing supervision before allowing the patient to eat).
- Gastrointestinal ulcer prophylaxis, as appropriate.
- Take out indwelling urinary (Foley) catheter as soon as possible.
- Monitor platelet counts if on heparin to watch for heparin-induced thrombocytopenia (HIT).

The following issues must be addressed daily:

- Is the patient neurologically stable or improving?
- Hydration:
  - Avoid dehydration of dysphagic patients with limited oral intake.
  - Avoid diuretics in patients receiving IV fluids.
- Is the patient medically stable (e.g., congestive heart failure, infection)?
- Is the blood pressure coming down slowly?
- Is the patient eating safely?
- Is the patient comfortable and sleeping well?
  - Ask yourself why the patient still gets blood drawn every morning for blood count, chemistry, calcium . . .
- What is the mechanism of the stroke?
  - Is the work-up appropriate and complete?

- What are we doing to prevent another stroke?
  - Ask yourself why the patient is not on antiplatelets, statins, ACE inhibitors – because most patients on the stroke service should be (except people with ICH or on anticoagulation).
- What are we doing to promote recovery?
- What are we doing to prevent complications from the stroke?
  - Don't forget DVT prophylaxis.
  - Ask yourself why the patient still has a Foley catheter and IV fluids if he or she is being discharged soon.
- What is the disposition?
- Think about disposition early:
  - Consult physical therapy, occupational therapy, speech therapy, and rehabilitation.
  - Contact primary care provider for follow-up.
  - Arrange home health care if indicated.

DRUG THERAPY IN THE FIRST 72 HOURS

The following are those most commonly started in our stroke unit:
- Antiplatelets:
  - Aspirin 81–325 mg once daily

  or
  - Clopidogrel (Plavix) 75 mg PO once daily, sometimes following a 300 mg load

  or
  - Both aspirin and clopidogrel

  or
  - Ticagrelor (60 mg PO bid) instead of clopidogrel if clopidogrel-resistant
  - Aspirin 25 mg/dipyridamole 200 mg extended-release (Aggrenox/Asasantin) twice daily

- DVT prophylaxis:
  - Heparin 5000 units SC every 8–12 hours

  or
  - Enoxaparin (Lovenox, Clexane) 40 mg SC once daily or 30 mg SC every 12 hours

  or
  - Dalteparin (Fragmin) 5000 units SC once daily
  - Sequential compression devices (non-drug)
- Anticoagulants for cardioembolic stroke:
  - Weight-adjusted heparin
  - Warfarin (Coumadin) (start with 5–10 mg PO qd)
  - Dabigatran (Pradaxa) 150 mg PO bid (adjust for renal insufficiency)
  - Rivaroxaban (Xarelto) 20 mg PO qd (adjust for renal insufficiency)
  - Apixaban (Eliquis) 5 mg PO bid (adjust for renal insufficiency, age, and weight)
  - Edoxaban (Svaysa) 60 mg PO qd (adjust for renal insufficiency)
- Insulin if needed.
- Temperature control with acetaminophen if needed.
- HMG CoA reductase inhibitors (statins) with goal of LDL < 70 mg/dL. It is important to make sure patients already taking statins continue to do so, even if it means placing a nasogastric tube to accomplish this.
- Oral antihypertensive agents:
  - ACE inhibitors:
    - Lisinopril (Prinivil, Zestril) 2.5–40 mg daily
    - Ramipril (Altace) starting at 2.5–5 mg daily; target 10 mg PO daily
  - Angiotensin II receptor blockers (ARBs):
    - Losartan (Cozaar) 25–100 mg daily
  - Diuretics:
    - Hydrochlorothiazide (HCTZ), chlorthalidone (Hygroton) 12.5–25 mg daily

- Beta-blockers:
  - Metoprolol (Lopressor, Toprol) 25–450 mg daily
- Calcium channel blockers:
  - Amlodipine (Norvasc) 5–10 mg daily
  - Nifedipine 30–90 mg daily

■ Recovery and Rehabilitation

See also Chapters 14, 15, and 16 on organization of stroke care, rehabilitation, and transition to outpatient management.

Physical therapy (PT), occupational therapy (OT), and speech therapy (ST) should get involved early.

Patients who are eating (after swallowing assessment by ST) are happy patients, and this also makes family members happy.

The sooner you get the patient and family involved in the process of recovery and rehabilitation the earlier you will be able to begin working on placement at the appropriate location (home, rehabilitation, skilled nursing facility [SNF], nursing home, or long-term acute care facility [LTAC]). The rehabilitation team is the key to determining disposition.

The only times when PT/OT would not be involved early is when the patient is obtunded or needs to lie flat in bed in an attempt to maximize cerebral perfusion. It is very important to get the patient mobilized with an out-of-bed (OOB) order (e.g., out of bed with meals, with PT, etc.). Mobilization also prevents complications.

■ Ischemic Stroke Outcome

Outcome after stroke depends on stroke severity, size, mechanism, age, premorbid functional status, whether and when the patient received tPA or EVT, and whether the patient is cared for in a stroke unit.

MORTALITY

Overall[8,9]

- ~30% mortality in the first year
- 40–50% in 5 years

From Medicare Database (Age ≥ 65 Years)[10]

- After surviving an ischemic stroke hospitalization, 26.4% mortality in 1 year, 60% mortality after 5 years
- After surviving a TIA hospitalization, 15% mortality in 1 year, 50% mortality in 5 years

DISABILITY

More importantly than mortality, patients and families are usually anxious to know the likely functional outcome. This is very difficult to predict in the first few days in an individual patient. It is best to offer a range from "worst case" to "best case" scenarios.

Table 3.2 shows outcome data based on ischemic stroke subtype, as determined by the extent of arterial occlusion, i.e., total, partial, or lacunar.

AT PATIENT DISCHARGE

Be sure you have determined or done the following:
- What is the stroke location and mechanism?
- What strategies are we using to prevent another stroke?
- Is the patient on any antihypertensives, in particular an ACE inhibitor?
- Is the patient on antiplatelets (e.g., aspirin, aspirin/dipyridamole, or clopidogrel)?
- Is the patient's LDL > 70 mg/dL, and if so, is he or she on a statin?

Table 3.2 Ischemic stroke outcomes from a population-based study in Australia

	Dead	Disabled	Non-disabled	Alive, not assessed
Total anterior circulation infarction (TACI)				
3 months	56%	29%	0%	15%
1 year	62%	24%	3%	12%
Partial anterior circulation infarction (PACI)				
3 months	13%	36%	24%	28%
1 year	25%	29%	24%	22%
Posterior circulation infarction (POCI)				
3 months	16%	20%	27%	38%
1 year	24%	22%	22%	31%
Lacunar infarction (LACI)				
3 months	8%	24%	31%	37%
1 year	8%	24%	31%	37%
Total				
3 months	20%	29%	22%	30%
1 year	31%	23%	23%	23%

Source: Dewey HM, Sturm J, Donnan GA, *et al.* Incidence and outcome of subtypes of ischaemic stroke: initial results from the North East Melbourne stroke incidence study (NEMESIS) *Cerebrovasc Dis* 2003; 15: 133–139.[11] Reproduced with permission from S. Karger A G, Basel.

- Get rid of unnecessary drugs.
- Is the follow-up plan established? If the patient is discharged on warfarin, who will be following the INR? This is critically important to communicate to the primary care providers as they are the ones who will be managing the risk factors of anticoagulation on a long-term basis.
- It is important to convey the mechanism of stroke and treatment recommendations to the primary care provider who will assume the primary responsibility for management of the patient on discharge.
- Write a discharge summary that includes the above thought processes.

■ General Timeline

The following is a general timeline for the care of stroke patients. It is influenced by the severity of the stroke, extent of diagnostic work-up necessary to determine etiology, ability to swallow, and amount of early recovery. The goal is to get patients discharged from acute hospitalization as quickly and as safely as possible.

- Stroke unit for 1–3 days.
- Then to the general ward to finish work-up and disposition determination.
- Discharge by day 2–5.

References

1. Powers WJ, Rabinstein AA, Ackerson T, *et al.*; American Heart Association Stroke Council. 2018 guidelines for the early management of patients with acute ischemic stroke: a guideline for healthcare professionals from the American Heart Association/American Stroke Association. *Stroke* 2018; 49: e46–e110.

2. European Stroke Organisation (ESO) Executive Committee, ESO Writing Committee. Guidelines for management of ischaemic stroke and transient ischaemic attack 2008. *Cerebrovasc Dis* 2008; 25: 457–507.

3. Anderson CS, Arima H, Lavados P, *et al.* HeadPoST Investigators and Coordinators. Cluster-randomized, crossover trial of head positioning in acute stroke. *N Engl J Med* 2017; 376: 2437–2447.

4. Hallevi H, Albright KC, Martin-Schild S, *et al.* Anticoagulation after cardioembolic stroke: to bridge or not to bridge? *Arch Neurol* 2008; 65: 1169–1173. doi:10.1001/archneur.65.9.noc70105.

5. Johnston KC, Bruno A, Pauls Q, *et al.*; Neurological Emergencies Treatment Trials Network and the SHINE Trial Investigators. Intensive vs standard treatment of hyperglycemia and functional outcome in patients with acute ischemic stroke: the SHINE Randomized Clinical Trial. *JAMA* 2019; 322: 326–335. doi: 10.1001/jama.2019.9346.

6. Albers GW, Amarenco P, Easton JD, Sacco RL, Teal P. Antithrombotic and thrombolytic therapy for ischemic stroke: the Seventh ACCP Conference on Antithrombotic and Thrombolytic Therapy. *Chest* 2004; 126 (3 suppl): 483S–512S.

7. Adams HP, Bendixen BH, Kappelle LJ, *et al.* Classification of subtype of acute ischemic stroke: definitions for use in a multicenter clinical trial. TOAST. Trial of Org 10172 in Acute Stroke Treatment. *Stroke* 1993; 24: 35–41.

8. Petty GW, Brown RD, Whisnant JP, *et al.* Survival and recurrence after first cerebral infarction: a population-based study in Rochester, Minnesota, 1975 through 1989. *Neurology* 1998; 50: 208–216.

9. Hartmann A, Rundek T, Mast H, *et al.* Mortality and causes of death after first ischemic stroke: the Northern Manhattan Stroke Study. *Neurology* 2001; 57: 2000–2005.

10. Bravata DM, Ho SY, Brass LM, *et al.* Long-term mortality in cerebrovascular disease. *Stroke* 2003; 34: 699–704.

11. Dewey HM, Sturm J, Donnan GA, *et al.* Incidence and outcome of subtypes of ischaemic stroke: initial results from the North East Melbourne stroke incidence study (NEMESIS). *Cerebrovasc Dis* 2003; 15: 133–139.

4

Stroke Radiology

■ Computed Tomography

Non-contrast CT (NCCT) of the head remains the standard procedure for the initial evaluation of stroke.

In the emergent initial evaluation of an acute stroke patient in the emergency department, NCCT remains the imaging modality utilized in most hospitals worldwide, with the exception of a few centers that have dedicated MRI capabilities for stroke. NCCT has the advantages of being widely available, relatively inexpensive, and fast to perform,[1] but the disadvantages of radiation exposure and not being able to exclude stroke mimics such as complicated migraine and peripheral vertigo, as compared to MRI. The clinical presentation of a patient with an intracerebral hemorrhage can be indistinguishable from that of an ischemic stroke. An NCCT must be performed prior to initiating IV thrombolytic therapy for acute ischemic stroke in order to rule out intracranial hemorrhage. NCCT should be performed within 20 minutes of the patient's arrival in the emergency department (ED) in order to expedite potential treatment with IV thrombolysis and/or endovascular thrombectomy (EVT) for ischemic stroke patients.

NCCT can also be utilized to determine whether an ischemic stroke is hyperacute (onset to 6 hours), acute (6 to 24 hours), subacute (24 hours to weeks) or chronic (weeks to months). In the first 6 hours from stroke onset, subtle early ischemic changes (EICs) appear first without hypodensity and represent ischemic tissue that is not yet infarcted, and thus amenable to IV thrombolysis. Later, as the infarction becomes irreversible, cytotoxic cerebral edema appears and the EICs appear as hypodense areas.[2] Detection of subtle EICs on NCCT generally requires the specialized training of a vascular neurologist or neuroradiologist. Presence of EICs should not be used to exclude patients from treatment with IV thrombolysis who meet the other inclusion and exclusion criteria.[3,4]

ACUTE ISCHEMIC APPEARANCES (GENERAL GUIDELINES)

- < 6 hours: no change in appearance
- *or*
- > 1.5 hours: loss of gray–white differentiation
- > 3 hours: hypodensity
- > 6 hours: swelling
- > weeks: ex-vacuo changes

WINDOW WIDTH AND LEVEL (WW/WL) FOR EARLY CT

The standard brain view on CT is set around 90/40. A setting of 40/40 may give high contrast of brain parenchyma to demonstrate the early ischemic signs more easily.

ASPECTS (ALBERTA STROKE PROGRAMME EARLY CT SCORE)

ASPECTS is scoring system that increases the reliability of detecting early CT changes in MCA territory infarction in the first few hours of ischemic stroke (Figure 4.1).[5]

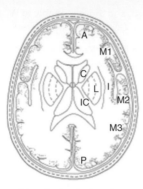 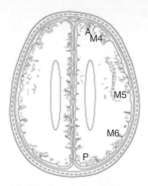

(a) at the level of basal ganglia and thalamus

(a) at the level just rostral to basal ganglia

10 regions of interest	
At the level of basal ganglia and thalamus	**At the level just rostral to basal ganglia**
C = caudate	
L = lentiform nuclei	
IC = internal capsule	
I = insular cortex	
M1 = anterior MCA cortex	M4 (superior to M1)
M2 = MCA cortex lateral to insula	M5 (superior to M2)
M3 = posterior MCA cortex	M6 (superior to M3)

Figure 4.1 ASPECTS template. (A black and white version of this figure will appear in some formats. For the color version, please refer to the plate section.)
Source: Barber PA, Demchuk AM, Zhang J, Buchan AM. Validity and reliability of a quantitative computed tomography score in predicting outcome of hyperacute stroke before thrombolytic therapy. ASPECTS Study Group. Alberta Stroke Programme Early CT Score. *Lancet* 2000; 355: 1670–1674.[5] Reproduced with permission from Elsevier.

Non-contrast head CT scans are interpreted at two levels:

1. at the level of the basal ganglia and thalamus
2. at the level just rostral to the basal ganglia

ACUTE HEMORRHAGE (EXTRAVASATED BLOOD)

This appears hyperdense (bright) on non-contrast CT at 40–60 Hounsfield units (HU). In the first few hours, the intensity may increase to 60–80 HUs. Intensity attenuates with time at a rate of ~0.7–1.5 HU/day.

The severity of hemorrhagic transformation into an ischemic stroke is classified according the ECASS trials as hemorrhagic infarction types 1 and 2 (HI-1, HI-2) and parenchymal hemorrhage types 1 and 2 (PH-1, PH-2) (Figures 4.2 and 7.5).[6–8]

■ Head CT with Contrast

CT ANGIOGRAPHY

CT angiography (CTA) of the head and neck with contrast is the mainstay for evaluating most acute stroke patients for the presence of a large-vessel occlusion (LVO) who may be candidates for EVT with mechanical thrombectomy. By current guidelines, all patients with a clinical presentation consistent with acute ischemic stroke with a premorbid modified Rankin scale (mRS) score of 0–1 (little or no disability at baseline), NIHSS of ≥ 6, who present within 6 hours of symptom onset, and an ASPECTS score of ≥ 6 should be considered potential EVT candidates and should therefore have CTA done at the same time as NCCT.[10] Performing CTA, however, should not delay the administration of IV thrombolysis, and therefore systems should be in place to initiate an IV tPA bolus and drip in the CT scanner suite while the CT technician sets up the contrast injection for CTA.

- Involves IV bolus of contrast, and imaging the arteries quickly during first pass of contrast.
- Allows visualization of vessels or lack thereof (occlusion, stenosis, AVM, aneurysms).

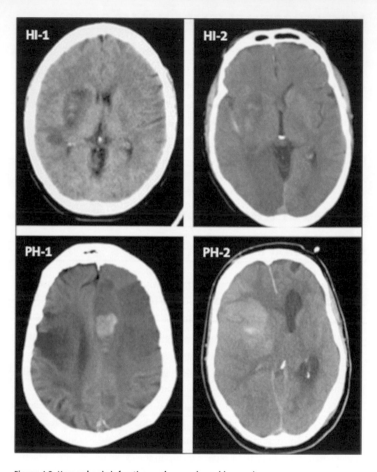

Figure 4.2 Hemorrhagic infarction and parenchymal hemorrhage.
Source: Álvarez-Sabín J, Maisterra O, Santamarina E, Kase CS. Factors influencing haemorrhagic transformation in ischaemic stroke. *Lancet Neurol* 2013; 12: 689–705.[9] Reproduced with permission from Elsevier.

- Requirements:
  - adequate renal function because the contrast bolus is larger than usual
  - good IV access, usually 18 gauge (you don't want contrast in soft tissues!)
- CT viewing window width/level at 800/100 may be best to visualize the arteries next to bones.
- Now done along with NCCT to identify arterial occlusion of major arteries and to plan endovascular therapies.

STANDARD HEAD CT WITH CONTRAST

Allows evaluation for stroke mimics by detecting blood–brain barrier breakdown:
- Tumor, infection, inflammation, etc.
- Rarely used in isolation in current clinical practice.

CT PERFUSION

Using an additional contrast bolus, CT perfusion (CTP) demonstrates which areas of the brain are receiving inadequate blood flow at the time of an acute ischemic stroke. CTP maps are increasingly being utilized in the acute setting to distinguish salvageable brain tissue (the "ischemic penumbra") from the irreversibly damaged tissue (the "core infarct"). The use of CTP to select patients who may be amenable to reperfusion with EVT in an extended time window is discussed in Chapter 6.

The most commonly used CTP parameters are:
- **CBV (cerebral blood volume)** – volume of blood per 100 g of brain in an imaging voxel. If the CBV is low, the brain tissue is considered to be irreversibly damaged ("core"). If the CBV is normal or high then this brain tissue is thought to be salvageable ("penumbra").

- **CBF (cerebral blood flow)** – volume of blood passing through 100 g of brain per minute. If the CBF is very low the brain tissue is irreversibly damaged. CBF may be slightly reduced in the penumbra.
- **MTT (mean transit time)** – average time it takes contrast bolus to move through a volume of brain in seconds. Both the core infarct and ischemic penumbra will have prolonged MTT in the setting of acute ischemic stroke.
- **TTP (time to peak)** – time in seconds from start of contrast injection to maximal enhancement of brain tissue.
- **T_{max} (maximum of the tissue residue function)** – similar to TTP, time in seconds for contrast bolus to perfuse brain tissue.[11]

Normal perfusion parameters are:

- gray matter
  - CBF: 60 mL/100 g/min
  - CBV: 4 mL/100 g
  - MTT: 4 s
- white matter
  - CBF: 25 mL/100 g/min
  - CBV: 2 mL/100 g
  - MTT: 4.8 s

RAPID (Rapid Processing of Perfusion and Diffusion) Software (Figure 4.3)

- CBF < 30% volume = critically hypoperfused, estimated as "core infarct."
- T_{max} > 6 seconds = severely hypoperfused, estimated as "ischemic penumbra."
- Mismatch ratio = ratio of volume of "penumbra" (T_{max} > 6 seconds) shown in green to volume of "core" (CBF < 30%) shown in pink, with a ratio of 1.8 found to indicate a favorable target for reperfusion.
- Used in DEFUSE 3 and DAWN trials to select extended window endovascular patients.[12,13]

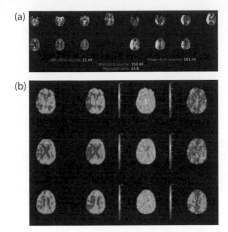

Figure 4.3 RAPID map. (a) Cerebral blood flow (CBF) < 30% (shown in pink on the left) represents a core infarct of 11 mL in a patient with a right middle cerebral artery (MCA) occlusion in the 6–24-hour window. The maximum of the tissue residue function (T_{max}) > 6 seconds (shown in green on the right) represents an ischemic penumbra of 161 mL. The mismatch volume is 150 mL, and the mismatch ratio is 14.6. (b) From left to right, the cerebral blood volume (CBV), CBF, mean transit time (MTT), and T_{max} are shown, demonstrating low blood volume in a small area of the right MCA territory with a much larger area at risk for infarction.

For further information, see: Albers GW. Use of imaging to select patients for late window endovascular therapy. *Stroke* 2018; 49: 2256–2260.[14] (A black and white version of this figure will appear in some formats. For the color version, please refer to the plate section.)

HOW TO TRY TO PREVENT CONTRAST-INDUCED ACUTE KIDNEY INJURY

- Hydration is the key to prevention of contrast-induced acute kidney injury.
- For high-risk patients (glomerular filtration rate [GFR] < 60, age > 75, sepsis, heart failure) consider intravenous 0.9% sodium chloride at a rate of 1 mL/kg/h for 12 hours before and after giving the contrast, whenever possible.

- Avoid nephrotoxic agents (NSAIDs, aminoglycosides).[15,16]
- Results of the Prevention of Serious Adverse Events Following Angiography (PRESERVE) trial demonstrated *no benefit* of periprocedural intravenous sodium bicarbonate or oral acetylcysteine over intravenous isotonic sodium chloride in prevention of contrast-induced acute kidney injury.[17]

■ Magnetic Resonance Imaging

EXCLUDING STROKE MIMICS

MRI is used as the primary screening modality for acute stroke treatment decision-making in the ED in only a small number of centers worldwide. However, MRI can be helpful in excluding stroke mimics such as peripheral vertigo and migraine with aura by demonstrating restricted diffusion consistent with acute infarct on diffusion-weighted imaging (DWI) sequences.

WAKE-UP STROKE

MRI brain can be used to select patients whose stroke symptoms are noted upon waking, and who may be eligible for tPA treatment beyond 4.5 hours from their last known normal time. Abnormal signals on FLAIR reflecting irreversible infarction begin to appear about 4–5 hours after stroke onset. In the WAKE-UP trial, patients who had restricted diffusion on DWI but no FLAIR sequence changes were potentially eligible for tPA treatment.[18] There seems to be a benefit of tPA treatment in selected wake-up stroke patients based on imaging, with a number needed to treat (NNT) of 9 (see Chapter 5).

DETERMINING STROKE ETIOLOGY

Although MRI of the brain is not generally feasible to perform in the hyperacute evaluation phase of a stroke patient, it can be helpful in determining etiology for both ischemic and hemorrhagic stroke patients.

In ischemic stroke, a cardioembolic etiology may be suggested by acute infarcts in multiple vascular territories or a cortical wedge-shaped infarction.[19]

Moreover, small infarcts that occur at the border of two vascular territories, so-called "borderzone" or "watershed" infarcts, may suggest a large-artery stenosis and stroke resulting from relative cerebral hypoperfusion through that narrowed artery.

In hemorrhagic stroke, the presence of cortical superficial siderosis and cortical microbleeds, along with a lobar intracerebral hemorrhage, would be suggestive of cerebral amyloid angiopathy as the etiology. Use of the modified Boston criteria may be helpful in categorizing the probability of cerebral amyloid angiopathy (CAA) as ICH etiology, based on neuroimaging findings.[20]

Magnetic resonance angiography (MRA) of the head and neck using a time-of-flight technique without contrast can be utilized instead of CTA in patients who cannot have a CT-based study performed, such as those who are pregnant, have a true contrast allergy, or cannot safely receive IV contrast because of advanced kidney disease.

■ MRI Sequences

Please refer to a more detailed text on MRI to explain all the physics of the different sequences. Here is a brief simplification of what each one looks like and what they are used for.

T1-WEIGHTED SEQUENCE

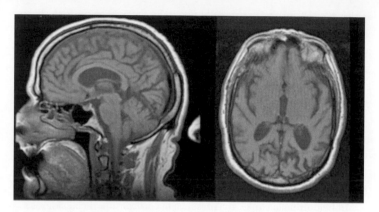

Figure 4.4 T1-weighted sequence (usually in axial and sagittal sections).

How to Identify

- Usually looks pale and bland.
- It looks the "most similar to CT."
- It appears exactly how you would expect the brain to look: cerebrospinal fluid is black; gray matter is gray; white matter is white.

Use

- Good for anatomy.
- Compare to T1 with contrast for leakage across blood–brain barrier.

T2-WEIGHTED SEQUENCE

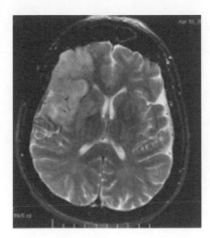

Figure 4.5 T2-weighted sequence.

How to Identify

- Exactly the opposite of how you would expect the brain to look: cerebrospinal fluid is white; gray matter is light; white matter is dark.

Use

- Good for pathology, and to evaluate flow voids.
- White: cerebrospinal fluid, edema, ischemia, and most bad things.
- Dark: old blood.

FLAIR

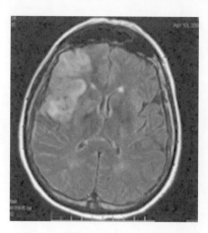

Figure 4.6 FLAIR (fluid-attenuated inversion recovery).

How to Identify

- Cerebrospinal fluid is dark; gray matter is light; white matter is dark.
- It is essentially T2 with the CSF made black.

Use

- Same as T2. It makes it easy to find pathology at CSF/brain junction (multiple sclerosis plaques, metastases, etc.) since on T2 it is sometimes difficult to tell what is CSF and what is pathological tissue.
- White: edema, infarction (begins to appear after 4–5 hours), and most bad things.
- Dark: CSF, old blood.

TIPS FOR IDENTIFYING T1, T2, AND FLAIR IMAGES

1. Look at CSF:
    a. If it is white, it is T2.
    b. If it is dark, go to step 2.
2. Look at gray and white matter:
    a. If it is normal, it is T1.
    b. If it is reversed, it is FLAIR.

DWI

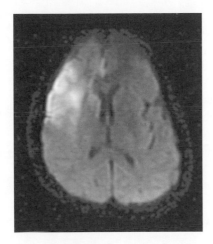

Figure 4.7 DWI (diffusion-weighted imaging).

How to Identify

• Uniformly gray grainy image.

Use

• Shows acute ischemia.

- White: acute ischemia (the proper term is restricted diffusion).
- Gray: everything else.
- With acute ischemic stroke, Na/K-ATPase fails and cells swell. Intracellular H_2O is less mobile than H_2O in the extracellular matrix. DWI is derived from the proton of the hydrogen atom.

Caution

- "T2 shine-through" – acute ischemia should be bright on DWI, dark on ADC (see below). Sometimes when T2 whiteness is strong in an old stroke, it "shines through" into DWI sequences. That's not acute stroke.
- Artifacts at air/bone interfaces – usually occur next to temporal bone and sinuses. These artifacts are usually symmetric and can be identified.
- Things that are not stroke – it turns out that many non-stroke things can appear bright on DWI. So look carefully for T2 shine-through and think whether the pattern is stroke-like (arterial distribution). Creutzfeldt–Jakob disease has cortical ribbons of DWI brightness. Wernicke encephalopathy shows restricted DWI symmetrically around the aqueduct and in mammillary bodies.
- DWI usually indicates irreversible ischemic damage, but in the first few hours, especially if not densely white (i.e., ADC not very low), DWI abnormalities can be reversed by reperfusion.

Time Course of DWI Intensity

- Maximal at 40 hours.
- Normalizes in 2 to several weeks.

ADC

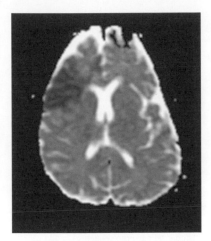

Figure 4.8 ADC (apparent diffusion coefficient).

How to Identify
• Grainy image with white cerebrospinal fluid.

Use
• Companion to DWI interpretation of acute ischemia.
• Dark on ADC in area where DWI is bright (white) is ischemia.
• One can think of it as "raw data" on DWI, except that ischemia is black. One can obtain quantitative measurements in the reduction in diffusion coefficient.

Time Course of ADC Intensity
• Maximal (dark) at 28 hours.
• Pseudonormalizes at 10 days, then bright.

MPGR/SWI

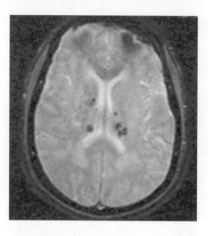

Figure 4.9 MPGR (multiplanar gradient recalled gradient-echo sequence) *or* SWI (susceptibility-weighted imaging).

How to Identify

- Grayish (it's hard by just looking).
- CSF in ventricles appears white.

Use

- Hemorrhages, whether new or old, appear dark.
- It is useful when looking for microhemorrhages such as those from amyloid angiopathy and cavernous malformations.
- One cannot measure the size of the hematoma on this image, since the signal is amplified and is bigger than the amount of blood.

PWI

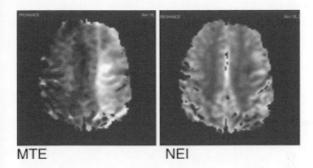

Figure 4.10 PWI (perfusion-weighted imaging).

How to Identify

There are two different sequences used:
- Mean time to enhancement (MTE) measures arrival time of bolus of dye. Areas of low cerebral perfusion look brighter (more light gray).
- Negative enhancement integral (NEI) measures cerebral blood volume (CBV). Areas of severe ischemia have reduced CBV and look dark. In mild ischemia, the vascular bed is dilated, CBV may be increased, and such regions will look bright.

Use

- PWI sequences measure cerebral blood flow.
- Look for a so-called "mismatch" between the changes on DWI, which are generally considered irreversible (but see fourth caution under DWI), and areas where there is a perfusion deficit on PWI. The areas of mismatch represent tissue at risk of infarction

("penumbra"). However, the best threshold for determining what perfusion defect represents truly threatened tissue that will die without reperfusion versus tissue that will survive ("benign oligemia") remains to be determined. The same is true in using CT perfusion to identify penumbra.

MRA

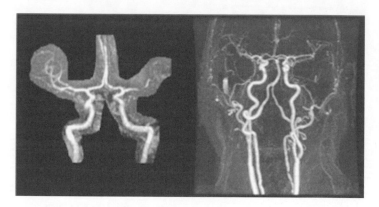

Figure 4.11 MRA (magnetic resonance angiography).

How to Identify
• You see the vessels.

Use
• Arterial stenosis: signal dropout more specific than appearance of stenosis.
• Aneurysms, vascular malformations (mostly AVM).

Caution

- There are a lot of artifacts in MRA images.
  - It's an artifact if there are consistent findings throughout a slice (e.g., image shifted).
- It shows flow rather than artery size, so in patent but low-flow states, MRA may falsely give the impression of occlusion.
- Some MRA sequences are flow-direction sensitive; reversed flow may appear as absent flow.
- MRA tends to overestimate stenosis.
- Ask a well-trained person to help with interpretation.
- If you are really interested in extracranial anatomy, especially aortic arch and vertebral origins, order MRA with contrast and speak to MRI technicians to ensure they know what you are looking for.

MRV

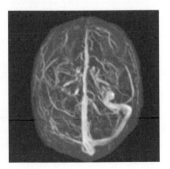

Figure 4.12 MRV (magnetic resonance venography).

How to Identify

• You see the veins.

Use

• Suspected venous sinus thrombosis. Suspect if hemorrhagic infarct, especially if bilateral, located high in convexity, associated with more edema than usual, or not fitting the usual arterial distribution of infarcts.

Caution

• Venous anatomy is variable.
• Especially troublesome is normal asymmetry of transverse sinuses. Ask for help in interpretation.

■ Usual Sequences Ordered for Acute Ischemic Stroke Patients

Estimated time 40 minutes.

• Sagittal T1
• Axial DWI
• Axial ADC
• Axial T2
• Axial T1
• Axial FLAIR
• Axial MPGR
• PWI (MTE and NEI)
• Axial T1 post-contrast (if PWI is done)
• Coronal T1 post-contrast (if PWI is done)
• MRA circle of Willis and neck

■ Abbreviated Protocol for Uncooperative Patients

Estimated time 10 minutes.

- DWI
- MRA circle of Willis and neck
- T2 or FLAIR

■ Usual Sequences Ordered for Acute ICH Patients

- Sagittal T1
- Axial T1
- Axial T2
- Axial FLAIR
- Axial MPGR
- Axial T1 post-contrast
- Coronal T1 post-contrast
- MRA circle of Willis
- MRV can be considered

MRI Findings in Brain Hemorrhage

Table 4.1 Sequential signal intensity (SI) changes of intracranial hemorrhage on MRI (1.5 T)

	Hyperacute hemorrhage	Acute hemorrhage	Early subacute hemorrhage	Late subacute hemorrhage	Chronic hemorrhage
What happens	Blood leaves the vascular system (extravasation)	Deoxygenation with formation of deoxy-Hb	Clot retraction and deoxy-Hb is oxidized to met-Hb	Cell lysis (membrane disruption)	Macrophages digest the clot
Time frame	< 12 h	Hours to days (weeks in center of hematoma)	A few days	4–7 days to 1 month	Weeks to years
Red blood cells intact	Erythrocytes	Intact, but hypoxic erythrocytes	Still intact, severely hypoxic	Lysis (solution of lysed cells)	Gone; encephalomalacia with proteinaceous fluid
State of Hb	Intracellular oxy-Hb	Intracellular deoxy-Hb	Intracellular met-Hb (first at periphery of clot)	Extracellular met-Hb	Hemosiderin (insoluble) and ferritin (water soluble)
T1-weighted images	$\approx$ or $\downarrow$	$\approx$ (or $\downarrow$)	$\uparrow\uparrow$	$\uparrow\uparrow$	$\approx$ or $\downarrow$
T2-weighted images	$\uparrow$ (high water content)	$\downarrow$ T2 PRE (susceptibility effect)	$\downarrow\downarrow$ T2 PRE (susceptibility effect)	$\uparrow\uparrow$ No T2 PRE (loss of compartmentalization)	$\downarrow\downarrow$ T2 PRE (susceptibility effect)

Hb, hemoglobin; T2 PRE, T2-proton relaxation enhancement; $\approx$, isointense relative to normal gray matter; $\uparrow$, increased SI (signal intensity) relative to normal gray matter; $\downarrow$, decreased SI relative to normal gray matter; $\downarrow\downarrow$, markedly decreased SI relative to normal gray matter.

Adapted from: Parizel PM, Makkat S, Van Miert E, *et al.* Intracranial hemorrhage: principles of CT and MRI interpretation. *Eur Radiol* 2001; 11: 1770–1783.[21] Reproduced with permission from Springer Science and Business Media.

■ Cerebral Angiogram

Diagnostic cerebral angiogram or digital subtraction angiography (DSA) is a catheter-based, fluoroscopy-guided imaging modality that is the gold standard for blood vessel imaging in acute ischemic stroke and for the evaluation of underlying vascular malformations in hemorrhagic stroke. For additional information regarding DSA please see Chapter 6 (*Endovascular Therapy*) and Chapter 12 (*Intracerebral Hemorrhage*).

■ Diffusion Tensor Imaging

Diffusion tensor imaging (DTI) is primarily used in research, and not in the clinical care of acute stroke patients. DTI tractography generates three-dimensional maps that show the organization and connectivity of white-matter tracts. There is early evidence to suggest that DTI may be utilized to predict Wallerian degeneration of the corticospinal tracts and therefore functional outcome.

References

1. Hand P, Wardlaw J, Rowat AM, *et al.* Magnetic resonance brain imaging in patients with acute stroke: feasibility and patient-related difficulties. *J Neurology Neurosurg Psychiatry* 2005; 76: 1525–1527.

2. von Kummer R, Bourquain H, Bastianello S, *et al.* Early prediction of irreversible brain damage after ischemic stroke at CT. *Radiology* 2001; 219: 95–100.

3. IST-3 Collaborative Group. Association between brain imaging signs, early and late outcomes, and response to intravenous alteplase after acute ischaemic stroke in the third International Stroke Trial (IST-3): secondary analysis of a randomised controlled trial. *Lancet Neurol* 2015; 14: 485–496.

4. Charidimou A, Pasi M, Fiorelli M, *et al.* Leukoaraiosis, cerebral hemorrhage, and outcome after intravenous thrombolysis for acute ischemic stroke: a meta-analysis (v1). *Stroke* 2016; 47: 2364–2372.

5. Barber PA, Demchuk AM, Zhang J, Buchan AM. Validity and reliability of a quantitative computed tomography score in predicting outcome of hyperacute stroke before thrombolytic therapy. ASPECTS Study Group. Alberta Stroke Programme Early CT Score. *Lancet* 2000; 355: 1670–1674.

6. Hacke W, Kaste M, Fieschi C, *et al*. Intravenous thrombolysis with recombinant tissue plasminogen activator for acute hemispheric stroke: the European Cooperative Acute Stroke Study (ECASS). *JAMA* 1995; 274: 1017–1025.

7. Hacke W, Kaste M, Fieschi C, *et al*. Randomised double-blind placebo-controlled trial of thrombolytic therapy with intravenous alteplase in acute ischaemic stroke (ECASS II). *Lancet* 1998; 352: 1245–1251.

8. Hacke W, Kaste M, Bluhmki E, *et al*. Thrombolysis with alteplase 3 to 4·5 hours after acute ischemic stroke. *N Engl J Med* 2008; 359: 1317–1329.

9. Álvarez-Sabín J, Maisterra O, Santamarina E, Kase CS. Factors influencing haemorrhagic transformation in ischaemic stroke. *Lancet Neurol* 2013; 12: 689–705.

10. Powers WJ, Rabinstein AA, Ackerson T, *et al*.; American Heart Association Stroke Council. 2018 guidelines for the early management of patients with acute ischemic stroke: a guideline for healthcare professionals from the American Heart Association/American Stroke Association. *Stroke* 2018; 49: e46–e110.

11. Allmendinger AM, Tang ER, Lui YW, *et al*. Imaging of stroke. Part 1, perfusion CT: overview of imaging technique, interpretation pearls, and common pitfalls. *Am J Roentgenol* 2012; 198: 52–62.

12. Straka M, Albers GW, Bammer R. Real-time diffusion–perfusion mismatch analysis in acute stroke. *J Magn Reson Imaging* 2010; 32: 1024–1037.

13. Calamante F, Christensen S, Desmond PM, *et al*. The physiological significance of the time-to-maximum (Tmax) parameter in perfusion MRI. *Stroke* 2010; 41: 1169–1174.

14. Albers GW. Use of imaging to select patients for late window endovascular therapy. *Stroke* 2018; 49: 2256–2260.

15. Lewington A, MacTier R, Hoefield R, *et al*. Prevention of contrast induced acute kidney injury (CI-AKI) in adult patients on behalf of the Renal Association, British Cardiovascular Intervention Society and the Royal College of Radiologists. https://renal.org/wp-content/uploads/2017/06/Prevention_of_Contrast_Induced_Acute_Kidney_Injury_CI-AKI_In_Adult_Patients-1.pdf (accessed May 2019).

16. Mueller C, Buerkle G, Buettner HJ, *et al*. Prevention of contrast media associated nephropathy: randomised comparison of 2 hydration regimens in 1620 patients undergoing coronary angioplasty. *Arch Intern Med* 2002; 162: 329–336.

17. Weisbord SD, Gallagher M, Jneid H, *et al.*; PRESERVE Trial Group. Outcomes after angiography with sodium bicarbonate and acetylcysteine. *N Engl J Med* 2018; 378: 603–614.

18. Thomalla G, Simonsen CZ, Boutitie F, *et al.*; WAKE-UP Investigators. MRI-guided thrombolysis for stroke with unknown time of onset. *N Engl J Med* 2018; 379: 611–622. doi:10.1056/NEJMoa1804355.

19. Novotny V, Thomassen L, Waje-Andreassen U, Naess H. Acute cerebral infarcts in multiple arterial territories associated with cardioembolism. *Acta Neurolog Scand* 2017; 135: 346–351.

20. Greenberg SW, Charidimou A. Diagnosis of cerebral amyloid angiopathy: evolution of the Boston criteria. *Stroke* 2018; 49: 491–497.

21. Parizel PM, Makkat S, Van Miert E, *et al.* Intracranial hemorrhage: principles of CT and MRI interpretation. *Eur Radiol* 2001; 11: 1770–1783.

5

Intravenous Thrombolysis

The only treatment that has been proven to improve outcome after ischemic stroke is to reperfuse the brain by removing the arterial obstruction. All animal and clinical studies show that brain tissue exposed to the reduced blood flow inherent after an arterial occlusion dies quickly, in proportion to the reduction of flow. Brain tissue where there is the most profound reduction of flow (the ischemic "core") dies within minutes. In areas where flow is less severely reduced (the ischemic "penumbra"), tissue death occurs more gradually, dependent on the adequacy of collateral flow. The faster that normal flow can be re-established, the less tissue death and the less consequent disability occurs. This chapter deals with systemic thrombolysis. Endovascular thrombectomy is discussed in Chapter 6.

Intravenous tPA is the only FDA-approved medical therapy for acute ischemic stroke, based on the pivotal NINDS tPA Stroke Study.[1] Since its approval in 1996, the utilization of tPA has steadily increased worldwide. In the US, the thrombolysis rate of all strokes went from 4% in 2003 to 7% in 2011.[2]

The first and most important step in stroke treatment is to recognize that a stroke is occurring, which has been covered in the previous chapters. However, because acute ischemic stroke is a clinical diagnosis and there is no rapid laboratory test with high sensitivity and specificity to confirm its presence, treatment with tPA is often carried out in patients where the diagnosis is not certain. Reassuringly, treatment of stroke "mimics" rarely produces hemorrhagic complications.[3] In most series in experienced stroke centers, the stroke-mimic treatment rate is 10–20%, but no higher.

The second step then is appropriate selection of stroke patients for tPA. Intravenous tPA is indicated for acute ischemic strokes of all types, e.g. due to embolism from the heart or proximal arteries, or thrombosis of large or small intracranial arteries, of all degrees of severity, and with most comorbidities. But within this broad umbrella, patient selection is critical. If guidelines are followed, there are substantial benefits and the risks are minimized. On the other hand, if these are violated, then the risks begin to outweigh the benefits. Many of the original contraindications to IV tPA have been relaxed in light of accruing evidence of safety and benefit. This is reflected in the most recent guidelines[4] and alteplase package insert.[5] As a result, there is some variability in how strictly the published exclusion criteria are applied in practice. For the most part, the indications and contraindications we list below follow published guidelines. We have indicated beneath each guideline where we might allow some flexibility in interpreting these criteria. As a general rule of thumb, the less severe and disabling the stroke, the less likely we are to ignore relative contraindications, and vice versa.

The other critical step in tPA treatment is to administer the drug as quickly as possible. The most effective way to improve results with tPA is by administering the drug as soon as possible after symptom onset – "time is brain" – with best results occurring when treatment is started within 90 minutes of symptom onset. Gradually decreasing benefit is seen as time elapses up to 4.5 hours, so that all causes of treatment delay, including unnecessary diagnostic tests, should be identified and eliminated (Figure 5.1). A handful of studies are under way to assess whether the time window of tPA administration can safely be extended to patients presenting late or those with stroke symptoms upon awakening. We will cover this topic later in the chapter.

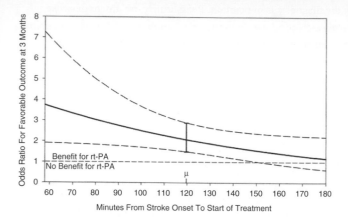

Figure 5.1 Model of favorable outcome at 3 months as a function of time to start of IV tPA treatment.

Source: Marler JR, Tilley BC, Lu M, *et al.* Early stroke treatment associated with better outcome. *Neurology* 2000; 55: 1649–1655.[6] Reproduced with permission.

■ tPA Indications

1. **Age 18 or older** – There are no data to guide treatment in children. However, there are case reports of older children being treated with tPA using adult criteria.

2. **Clinical diagnosis of ischemic stroke causing a measurable neurological deficit** – In most but not all cases, NIHSS ≥ 3. However, there is no absolute lower NIHSS cutoff, remembering that the NIHSS does not measure disability. We use the criterion, "Would the neurological deficit be at all disabling if it were to persist?"

3. **Onset of stroke symptoms well established to be less than 180 minutes (or 270 minutes [4.5 hours] in Europe and some US centers) before treatment would begin** – We have addressed the

importance of establishing the time of onset in Chapter 2. Intravenous tPA between 3 and 4.5 hours after stroke onset has been demonstrated to be effective in a randomized clinical trial in Europe, the ECASS III trial,[7] and is incorporated in the AHA guideline recommendations. It is approved in Europe but not yet approved by the FDA in the USA.

■ tPA Contraindications

STRONG CONTRAINDICATIONS

1. **Known history of intracranial hemorrhage** – The alteplase package insert recommends only to "use caution" in treating patients with recent ICH, but it remains an absolute contraindication in the AHA/ASA guidelines. We would treat a patient with a remote (> 3 months old) ICH as long as the cause of the bleeding was no longer present.

2. **Symptoms suggestive of subarachnoid hemorrhage** – However, in a patient with "the worst headache of my life," if careful reading of the CT shows no SAH, and the patient otherwise has a clinical presentation consistent with focal ischemic stroke, then treatment with tPA should be given.

3. **Any evidence of bleeding on the pretreatment head CT** – If there is *any* bleeding seen on the CT, the patient should not be treated. The CT should be carefully reviewed and any lesions suggestive of bleeding would exclude treatment. Remember that isodense subdural hematomas can be easily overlooked. It is uncertain whether patients with the parenchymal "microbleeds" often seen with amyloid angiopathy that are seen on gradient-echo MRI (and not CT) can be safely treated. The available data suggest that the risk of symptomatic ICH after tPA is increased and long-term functional outcome worse in patients who have > 10 cortical microbleeds on a baseline MRI. It is unclear whether the benefit of tPA in this patient population outweighs

the risk of bleeding. We do not recommend a screening MRI in patients prior to tPA, though it might be reasonable in a patient with a relatively minor stroke and strong suspicion of underlying amyloid angiopathy.

4. **Intracranial neoplasm, untreated arteriovenous malformation (AVM), or aneurysm that is at risk of bleeding** – If the patient has an aneurysm or AVM that has been surgically clipped or repaired more than 3 months ago, we would probably allow treatment, though, if quickly available, we might do a CTA first to confirm obliteration of the lesion. The current guidelines state that it is probably reasonable to treat patients with unsecured unruptured aneurysms < 10 mm in size. No recommendation is made about larger aneurysms. Untreated AVMs should not be treated. Many patients with benign brain tumors such as meningiomas have been treated without complications. However, patients with more aggressive parenchymal brain tumors such as gliomas or metastases should not be treated.

5. **Significant hypodensity or mass effect on pretreatment CT** – Early ischemic changes on the CT are not a contraindication. However, clearly demarcated hypodensity suggesting that the stroke is more than 3 hours old would argue against treatment. Mass effect with compression of the ventricle or midline structures would suggest a non-stroke etiology.

6. **Previous intracranial surgery, or serious head trauma within the past 3 months**.

7. **Sustained systolic blood pressure > 185 mmHg (with warning for > 175 mmHg, per the alteplase package insert), *or* sustained diastolic blood pressure > 110 mmHg** – Aggressive treatment is necessary to lower blood pressure to these levels (see comments on blood-pressure control, below).

8. **Active internal bleeding**.

9. **Received heparin within 48 hours AND has an elevated PTT**.

10. **Platelet count < 100 000**. A platelet count is not necessary unless there is a clinical suspicion of thrombocytopenia. The 100 000 level,

while in the guidelines, is arbitrary and it may be safe to treat patients with platelet counts of > 50 000 as long as there is no history of clinical bleeding. Again, stroke severity will play into this decision.

11. **INR > 1.7 or known bleeding diathesis** – We tend to be a little more conservative than published guidelines about the INR level that would allow treatment with IV tPA. In the NINDS trial, the cutoff used was a prothrombin time (PT) of 15 seconds. There is debate as to what INR level correlates with this level of PT. However, we know that increased bleeding occurs when patients treated with warfarin reach an INR of 1.7 or higher. In a patient with an INR of 1.6, we would consider omitting tPA and going for endovascular thrombectomy (EVT) if it is immediately available and the patient has an intracranial large-vessel occlusion (LVO). Even with these considerations, it should be emphasized that an INR is not required prior to treatment if the patient is not on warfarin or there is no reason to suspect abnormal liver function or coagulopathy.

12. **Known bleeding diathesis**.

13. **Use of direct thrombin inhibitors or factor Xa inhibitors within the last 48 hours or if coagulation tests are abnormal** (e.g., aPTT, INR, platelet count, ecarin clotting time, thrombin time, or appropriate factor Xa activity assays). There have been case reports where patients with acute ischemic stroke occurring within 48 hours of taking dabigatran are given the immediately acting reversal agent idarucizumab and then successfully and safely given tPA.[8] The same may be true with andexanet alpha for patients on Xa inhibitors now that it is available. However, more clinical experience with this practice is needed before it can be routinely recommended. Again, patients on direct thrombin inhibitors or Xa inhibitors might be better candidates for EVT if they also harbor an LVO.

14. **Suspected or known aortic arch dissection** – This should be considered in patients presenting with chest pain or hypotension.

15. **Suspected or known septic embolization/infective endocarditis** – Embolic cerebral infarcts from endocarditis may have a high rate of spontaneous hemorrhagic conversion. Thrombolysis in this setting is expected to have a higher hemorrhage rate.

RELATIVE CONTRAINDICATIONS

1. **Minor or rapidly improving symptoms** – This scenario presents one of the most difficult decisions in treating patients with tPA and is the second most frequent cause for non-treatment of otherwise eligible patients (the first is being outside the established time window of 3–4.5 hours from onset). Guidelines state not to treat a patient who is rapidly improving. However, many such patients recover substantially but are still left with a disabling deficit. Even patients with very mild strokes benefit from tPA treatment, and intracranial bleeding complications in such patients are very rare. Therefore, instead of automatically excluding all patients who are improving or have minor deficits, we would still treat the minor or improving patient whose deficit, at the time you are ready to treat, would be disabling if it persisted. The PRISMS trial, which was terminated early because of slow recruitment and was therefore underpowered, did not show any benefit in treating non-disabling minor strokes.[9]

2. **Ischemic stroke in the last 3 months** – The current guidelines recommend against treating with IV tPA in this population. The alteplase package insert removed the exclusion. Because the highest risk of stroke recurrence is within the first 3 months, it is common that patients present with this relative "contraindication." The risk of tPA treatment in these patients is creating hemorrhagic transformation of the previous stroke. Here in particular the severity of the previous and incident strokes, and the elapsed interval between them, is important. The smaller and more remote the previous stroke, and the more severe the incident stroke, the more likely we are to allow tPA treatment.

3. **Gastrointestinal or urinary tract hemorrhage within the last 21 days** – In some cases, we are not so rigid with regard to time intervals for GI and GU bleeding, allowing for clinical judgment based on the severity of the anticipated risk versus the possible benefit. For instance, one might be willing to treat a patient with a very severe stroke who has had some recent GI bleeding, knowing that this complication might occur, but also knowing that without treatment the outcome is likely to be very poor. This risk would be less acceptable in a patient with a milder stroke. The main caveat is that if the patient is actively bleeding, as evidenced by a low hemoglobin/hematocrit, that patient should not be treated. If you do treat a patient with risk of bleeding, then consultation with the appropriate surgical consultant who could help manage the hemorrhagic complication should be obtained at the time of treatment, in anticipation of, and not after, the complication occurs.

4. **Major surgery or serious extracranial trauma within previous 14 days** – again, severity of potential complications must be weighed against severity of the stroke. Obtaining a surgical consult prior to tPA administration is recommended.

5. **Arterial puncture at a non-compressible site, or lumbar puncture** – Guidelines state that tPA should not be given within 7 days of such punctures, but clinical judgment is necessary. Usually, 24 hours should be a sufficient interval if there is no evidence of an especially traumatic puncture.

6. **Seizure at the onset of stroke** – Patients with seizures were excluded from the initial studies of tPA because they made it difficult to assess how much of the neurological deficit was due to the seizure and how much due to the stroke. This is important when carrying out a clinical trial, but less important in clinical practice. If you are sure that a stroke has occurred that is causing a disabling deficit, even if the patient has had a seizure, it is appropriate to treat that patient if he or she qualifies by other criteria (particularly no evidence of head trauma with the

seizure, and no mass effect on CT). CTA showing arterial occlusion, or DWI showing acute ischemic damage, can help in this situation if either can be carried out quickly. CT perfusion showing hyperemia may also point to a seizure rather than a stroke.

7. **Blood glucose < 50 mg/dL or > 400 mg/dL** – A patient who remains symptomatic after a high or low glucose is treated and normalized need not be excluded.

8. **Hemorrhagic eye disorder, and other conditions likely to cause disability if bleeding occurs** – Recent ocular surgery such as for cataracts, and other minor surgery, are not necessarily contraindications. Judgment is needed. Treatment of a patient with some ocular conditions, such as a recently detached retina, might pose too great a risk of visual loss, especially if the stroke is relatively mild. The best course is to try to reach the specialist consultant and ask for an opinion about bleeding risk.

9. **Myocardial infarction in the previous 3 months** – Judgment should be utilized in interpreting this exclusion. Both the time interval from the MI and the severity of the MI should be taken into consideration. Per the guidelines, it is reasonable to treat recent NSTEMI and STEMI involving the right or inferior myocardium, whereas it *may* be reasonable to treat left anterior STEMI. The main risk here is hemorrhagic pericarditis and pericardial tamponade. This would certainly be a risk with a recent transmural MI or open-heart surgery, but a smaller MI, even if recent, would not be considered a contraindication. Concurrent acute ischemic stroke and acute MI is not a contraindication to tPA.

10. **Pregnancy** – The concern with the use of tPA in pregnancy is the risk of uterine bleeding, not a teratogenic effect (class C). Additionally, tPA is too large a molecule to cross the placenta. The benefit to the mother of using tPA, especially taking into consideration the severity of the stroke, must be weighed against the risk of uterine bleeding, especially in high-risk patients (e.g., placental abruption, intrapartum bleeding).

EVT might be an alternative but exposes the fetus to radiation. As a side note, tPA can probably be safely administered during lactation because it is broken down by the infant's GI tract and its large size does not allow it to cross the gut–blood barrier.

11. **Intracranial arterial dissection** – the efficacy and safety of tPA administration in the setting of a known or suspected intracranial arterial dissection are not well studied and remain unclear. It should not be given if there is any associated subarachnoid bleeding on the CT. Patients with extracranial dissection can be safely treated, since most strokes in this setting result from emboli to the intracranial arteries.

ADDITIONAL EXCLUSIONS FOR 3–4.5-HOUR TIME WINDOW

As a reminder, the FDA has not approved the use of tPA for acute ischemic strokes beyond 3 hours from the time the patient was last known well (LKW). In Europe, however, tPA is approved for the 3–4.5-hour time window, notwithstanding a few exclusions, and many medical centers in the USA will treat in this extended window. The following were exclusions in the ECASS III trial and were used to provide the basis for the EMA approval of tPA in the extended window. However, the current guidelines revised these points and many of them no longer constitute exclusions:

1. **Patients older than 80 years (no longer an exclusion)** – tPA administration is as safe and effective in elderly as in younger patients.
2. **Use of warfarin, regardless of INR (no longer an exclusion)** – tPA is beneficial and safe in patients with INR < 1.7 in the extended window, though the same caveats apply as for patients within 3 hours.
3. **Prior history of both stroke and diabetes (no longer an exclusion)** – This group of patients was seen as "poor responders" in a secondary analysis of prior trials and was not entered in the ECASS III study.

Subsequent registry and pooled analyses suggest that, while response may be less, they may still benefit.

4. **Severe stroke, such as baseline NIHSS > 25 or involvement of more than one-third of MCA territory on non-contrast CT (caution still needs to be exercised)** – In the later time window, with the diminishing benefit/risk ratio, severe strokes due to LVO are at low likelihood to benefit from tPA. Similarly, extensive early ischemic changes found on CT in this time window indicate too much established damage, and tPA should not be administered.

WAKE-UP STROKES, STROKES OF UNKNOWN TIME OF ONSET, AND PATIENTS BEYOND 4.5 HOURS

Up to a third of ischemic strokes occur during sleep. Uncertain time of onset is the reason why almost 25% of ischemic stroke patients are not considered eligible for IV tPA. It is likely that a proportion of these patients may still be within the 4.5-hour time window of tPA efficacy. Even in those who are beyond 4.5 hours, it is likely that a diminishing proportion with adequate collateral flow will still retain salvageable tissue.

Several studies have been done or are under way to establish the safety and benefit of treating these patients. These studies have used various degrees of advanced imaging to identify patients who may still have salvageable tissue.

1. **Wake-up or unknown-onset patients**
   - SAIL ON showed that it is safe to treat patients presenting within 4.5 hours of waking up as long as the initial NCCT does not contain ischemic changes that involve more than one-third of MCA territory.[10]
   - WAKE-UP was a randomized trial of tPA versus non-treatment in patients based on MRI showing presence of a responsible lesion on diffusion-weighted imaging but no FLAIR lesion (previous MRI data had

shown that FLAIR hyperintensities don't begin to appear until about 4.5 hours after stroke onset). The results were similar to those seen in patients treated within 4.5 hours based on NCCT – a highly significant increase in the chance of benefit balanced against an increased risk of bleeding, with overall benefit in favor of tPA.[11]

2. **Patients beyond 4.5 hours of LKW**

   - EXTEND recently showed that there is a benefit in treating patients who demonstrate salvageable penumbral tissue on perfusion imaging between 4.5 and 9 hours from LKW. For patients to be enrolled, the ischemic core volume had to be < 70 mL and the perfusion–ischemia mismatch ratio had to be > 1.2. CT perfusion or perfusion–diffusion MRI were used. The tPA group achieved the primary outcome of modified Rankin scale (mRS) 0–1 at 90 days with an adjusted risk ratio of 1.44 (95% CI 1.01–2.06, $p = 0.04$) compared to placebo. Symptomatic ICH occurred in 6.2% of the tPA group versus 0.9% in the placebo group, resulting in an adjusted risk ratio of 7.22 (95% CI 0.97–53.5, $p = 0.05$).[12]

   - MR WITNESS enrolled patients between 4.5 hours and 24 hours from LKW who could be treated within 4.5 hours of symptom discovery. It showed that tPA administration was safe in patients who were selected based on diffusion–FLAIR mismatch on MRI, i.e., presence of diffusion restriction and either minimal or no hyperintense changes on T2-weighted FLAIR images. However, efficacy of treatment could not be determined.[13]

   - EPITHET and DEFUSE 2 showed that stroke patients with onset time between 3 and 6 hours and with diffusion–perfusion mismatch (critically hypoperfused penumbra defined as $T_{max} > 6$ s) had significantly smaller infarcts and better reperfusion rates with IV tPA compared to placebo. Again, efficacy was not established.[14,15]

In summary, guidelines still do not support treating patients with tPA unless treatment can be definitely established within 4.5 hours of LKW. However, the bulk of data suggest that wake-up and unknown-onset patients can be treated with tPA safely if the NCCT scan is normal, and that treatment is likely to be most effective in those selected using advanced imaging, as was done in the WAKE-UP study. While we would treat selected patients based on these data, further study is needed to confirm the WAKE-UP data, and to determine if beneficial results can be accomplished using CT and CT perfusion as well as with MRI diffusion/FLAIR, which takes more time and is not available in many centers.

BLOOD-PRESSURE CONTROL

Blood-pressure control is very important to prevent complications (see Table 3.1). Before treatment, the goal is systolic < 185 mmHg and diastolic < 110 mmHg. Labetalol (Trandate, Normodyne) 10–20 mg IV or a nicardipine (Cardene) drip (start at 5 mg/h and titrate up to a maximum of 15 mg/h) may be given to lower the blood pressure. If SBP is > 200, we find it is always necessary to start nicardipine. If you are unable to keep the BP in the specified range with labetalol < 40 mg or nicardipine < 15 mg/h, the risk of hemorrhage is too high and the patient should not receive tPA. Blood-pressure control to SBP ≤ 180 during and after tPA administration is equally important, and BP should be checked every 15 minutes to make sure it stays under control. This is often difficult to accomplish in the busy ED setting where nurses have many other patients to manage, so rapid admission to a specialized stroke unit experienced in managing post-tPA patients should be a priority.

■ Procedure

FAST!

Remember: **time is brain**. Best results occur with treatment started within 2 hours of symptom onset. Door-to-needle time: goal is < 40 minutes, maximum is 60 minutes.

1. Check to make sure laboratory tests are sent immediately and ECG ordered (ordered, drawn, and sent within the first 5 minutes).
   • Glucose is the only blood test you need before treatment in most patients and can be obtained by fingerstick.
   • Send complete blood count (CBC) and platelets.
   • INR if the patient is on anticoagulants or coagulopathy is suspected. Some centers now have point-of-care INR. While not as accurate, it is probably sufficient.
   • Urine pregnancy test if appropriate.
2. Examine patient (within the next 5 minutes).
   • Establish clear time of onset.
   • Obtain pertinent historical details (e.g., past medical history, medications).
   • NIH Stroke Scale (Appendix 7).
   • Check blood pressure.
3. Obtain non-contrast head CT (maximum ED arrival to CT time should be 25–30 minutes).
4. Talk to patient and family to explain risks/benefits.
5. Obtain the patient's weight (if no bed scale, ask the patient or family member(s), or estimate).
   • If the patient weighs over 100 kg (220 lb) he/she will get the maximum dose and it is not important to figure out the exact weight.
6. Think again: go over indications/contraindications and lab and imaging results.

7. Check BP again.
8. Pre-therapy: two peripheral IV lines.
   - Do not place Foley catheter unless absolutely necessary.
   - ECG can be done after IV tPA is started.

DOSE

Alteplase

- 0.9 mg/kg up to a maximum of 90 mg total
- 10% given as IV bolus over 1 minute
- Remaining 90% infused over 1 hour

Because of perceived higher rates of bleeding risk in Asian patients, a large study (ENCHANTED) compared standard-dose tPA to a lower dose, 0.6 mg/kg with 15% given as a bolus (so that the bolus remained the same as with standard dose). The study enrolled comparable numbers of Asian and non-Asian patients. The results showed that the lower dose could not be proven to be non-inferior to standard-dose tPA, and that there was no difference between Asian and non-Asian patients. Nevertheless, lower-dose treatment is standard of care in some Asian countries. There was a significantly lower risk of spontaneous ICH with the lower dose of alteplase.[16]

Other Lytics

Tenecteplase (TNK, TNKase, Metalyse) has the theoretic advantage of being a more fibrin-specific thrombolytic compared to tPA, and it has a longer half-life so is given as a single bolus without an infusion. Several studies have compared various doses of TNK to tPA in tPA-eligible patients.

- Early studies of TNK. Relatively small dose escalation studies and randomized phase II studies suggested increased bleeding with TNK doses above 0.4 mg/kg, and comparable bleeding but no significant benefit for TNK over tPA at doses of 0.1–0.4 mg/kg.

- NOR-TEST was a randomized comparison of TNK 0.4 mg/kg bolus to standard-dose tPA in 1100 patients and found no difference in efficacy or bleeding with TNK.[17]

- EXTEND-IA TNK was limited to patients who were candidates for EVT, with standard-dose tPA or TNK 0.25 mg/kg bolus given as "bridging" therapy. It showed that TNK was not inferior to tPA. In fact, TNK was associated with higher reperfusion rates, no increased bleeding, and better 90-day functional outcomes in patients treated within 4.5 hours from LKW.[18]

- Further studies are under way testing TNK compared to tPA and, if comparable or superior efficacy is established, it is possible that because of its greater convenience it will gain increased use over the next few years. However, the best dose still needs to be established. For now, tPA is the only approved treatment for acute ischemic stroke.

Other drugs that may be given to patients with myocardial infarction may not be used for stroke. These include reteplase (Retavase) and streptokinase (Streptase). Make sure to double-check the name of the drug, because there are some hospitals that may not carry tPA. ED personnel may reach for one of the other thrombolytic drugs because of familiarity with their use in acute MI. Also, the dosing for stroke and acute MI is different.

■ Risks Versus Benefits of tPA

WHAT ARE THE BENEFITS OF tPA THERAPY?

1. The percentage of patients with excellent outcome (Rankin 0–1) is increased by about 15% absolute or 50% relative when treated early (within 3 hours), 7% absolute or 12% relative when treated late (3–4.5 hours). The percentage with bad outcome (dead or

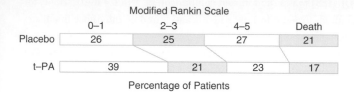

Figure 5.2 Three-month outcome in NINDS tPA study by modified Rankin scale (mRS). (A black and white version of this figure will appear in some formats. For the color version, please refer to the plate section).
Source: National Institute of Neurological Disorders and Stroke rt-PA Stroke Study Group. Tissue plasminogen activator for acute ischemic stroke. *N Engl J Med* 1995; 333: 1581–1587.[1] Reproduced with permission.

Rankin 4–5) is reduced, even if you include the patients who bleed (Figure 5.2).

2. The odds ratio of good outcome is 1.7 (95% CI 1.2–2.6) when treated early and 1.3 (95% CI 1.0–1.7) when treated late.

3. Patients treated with tPA within 3 hours of onset are 30–50% more likely (relative risk increase) to have minimal or no disability at 3 months. The benefit is diminished with treatment in the 3–4.5-hour window, with a 16% increase in the chance of having minimal or no disability at 3 months.

4. NNT (number needed to treat) = 3 to result in 1 patient with better outcome than if not treated when treated within 3 hours, 6 to result in 1 patient with better outcome when treated in the 3–4.5-hour window, 8 to result in 1 patient with complete recovery when treated within 3 hours.

5. NNH (number needed to harm) = 33 to result in 1 patient with worse outcome than if not treated when treated within 3 hours, 37 to result in 1 patient with worse outcome when treated in the 3–4.5-hour window.

WHO BENEFITS?

1. All stroke subtypes benefit.
2. Both mild (NIHSS ≤ 7) and severe (NIHSS ≥ 15) stroke patients benefit.
3. Elderly as well as young patients benefit, but there are few data in the pediatric population.
4. Patients with early ischemic changes on CT still benefit if they meet all other criteria when treated within 3 hours of onset.
5. Time to treatment is the key to an improved chance of recovery.[6] Patients treated earlier are more likely to respond than those treated at the end of the 3-hour window. Therefore, time is brain!

WHAT ARE THE RISKS OF tPA THERAPY?

1. **Symptomatic intracranial hemorrhage** rate 6.4% (i.e., 1 in 16; 95% CI 3.5–9.2%) versus 0.6% in placebo when treated early (within 3 hours), and 7.9% (i.e., 1 in 12) when treated during the expanded time window (3–4.5 hours). However, this is using the original definition of symptomatic hemorrhage, which was any bleeding on follow-up scan associated with neurological worsening even if the worsening was due to other factors such as the expected edema associated with the stroke. When more strict definitions of hemorrhage are used, such as hematoma occupying more than one-third of the infarcted region (parenchymal hemorrhage type 2, or PH-2), or PH-2 hemorrhage with 4-point deterioration on NIHSS (SITS-MOST), rates are much lower, in the range of 2–3%. Also, while there is progressively less benefit over the 4.5-hour time window for treatment, there is no increased risk of bleeding during that time window.
2. **Angioedema** – In a retrospective series, it was reported to occur at a rate of 5.1% (95% CI 2.3–9.5%),[19] but this is probably an overestimate

(see below for treatment options). Occurs more frequently in patients taking ACE inhibitors.

WHO IS MORE LIKELY TO BLEED?

1. Patients with more severe stroke.
2. Patients with extensive CT changes, BP above guidelines at time of treatment or afterwards, elevated glucose or temperature, and those of advanced age.
3. But even those with severe strokes, early CT changes, and advanced age show overall benefit with tPA treatment, even accounting for the chances of bleeding. This is because, without treatment, such patients are universally going to do poorly.[20,21]

■ tPA-Related Intracranial Hemorrhage: Management Protocol

Suspect intracranial hemorrhage if the patient develops severe headache, acute elevation in blood pressure, nausea, vomiting, or neurological deterioration.

1. Stop tPA infusion if still running.
2. Stabilize patient – airway, breathing, circulation (ABCs). Patient may need intubation if airway protection is needed.
3. Obtain STAT non-contrast head CT.
4. Reverse effect of tPA. Goal: fibrinogen level > 200 mg/dL with cryoprecipitate.
   a. Type and cross, INR, PTT, complete blood count.
   b. Check fibrinogen level immediately and every 6 hours.
   c. Give 10–20 units of cryoprecipitate before level returns (1 unit raises fibrinogen by 5–10 mg/dL; assume there is no fibrinogen and adjust dose when level is back).

d. Repeat cryoprecipitate if needed.

e. May use fresh frozen plasma (FFP) in case of no cryoprecipitate (1 unit of cryoprecipitate is made from 1 bag of FFP).

f. May give platelet concentrate if low.

g. Activated factor VII is untested in this situation, and should not be used.

h. Control BP to prevent expansion of hematoma. We recommend maintaining SBP < 160.

i. Neurosurgery should be called; however, surgery cannot be done until coagulopathy is corrected and is usually not indicated (see Chapter 12).

■ Oropharyngeal Angioedema: Management Protocol

1. Usually happens towards the end of the tPA infusion.

2. Repeatedly examine oropharynx, watching for edema (may be subtle swelling of lip or tongue just on one side).

3. If angioedema is suspected, discontinue the infusion, hold ACE inhibitor, immediately call for personnel experienced in intubation and airway management. Do not wait until airway obstruction occurs.

4. Choose from the following medication options:

   a. Epinephrine 0.5 mL via nebulizer or 0.3 mL of 0.1% solution subcutaneously (may repeat twice as tolerated).

   b. Diphenhydramine (Benadryl) 50 mg IV followed by 25 mg every 6 hours × 4 doses.

   c. Methylprednisolone (Solu-Medrol) 125 mg IV; may follow with 20–80 mg IV daily for 3–5 days depending on degree and course of angioedema.

   d. Famotidine 20 mg IV (or ranitidine 50 mg IV) followed by 20 mg IV (or ranitidine 50 mg IV) every 12 hours × 2 doses.

5. If further increase in oropharyngeal angioedema is seen, or if there is airway compromise:
   a. If tongue is edematous, but oral intubation is possible, perform urgent orotracheal intubation.
   b. If tongue is too edematous for orotracheal intubation, perform fiberoptic nasotracheal intubation.
   c. If there is severe stridor or impending airway obstruction, perform tracheostomy or cricothyrotomy and consider reversing tPA.
   d. Always resolves spontaneously within 24 hours without sequelae.

References

1. National Institute of Neurological Disorders and Stroke rt-PA Stroke Study Group. Tissue plasminogen activator for acute ischemic stroke. *N Engl J Med* 1995; 333: 1581–1587.
2. Schwamm LH, Ali SF, Reeves MJ, *et al.* Temporal trends in patient characteristics and treatment with intravenous thrombolysis among acute ischemic stroke patients at Get With The Guidelines-Stroke hospitals. *Circ Cardiovasc Qual Outcomes* 2013; 6: 543–549.
3. Chernyshev OY, Martin-Schild S, Albright KC, *et al.* Safety of tPA in stroke mimics and neuroimaging-negative cerebral ischemia. *Neurology* 2010; 74: 1340–1345.
4. Powers WJ, Rabinstein AA, Ackerson T, *et al.*; American Heart Association Stroke Council. 2018 guidelines for the early management of patients with acute ischemic stroke: a guideline for healthcare professionals from the American Heart Association/American Stroke Association. *Stroke* 2018; 49: e46–e110.
5. Demaerschalk BM, Kleindorfer DO, Adeoye OM, *et al.*; American Heart Association Stroke Council and Council on Epidemiology and Prevention. Scientific rationale for the inclusion and exclusion criteria for intravenous alteplase in acute ischemic stroke: a statement for healthcare professionals from the American Heart Association/American Stroke Association. *Stroke* 2016; 47: 581–641.
6. Marler JR, Tilley BC, Lu M, *et al.* Early stroke treatment associated with better outcome: the NINDS rt-PA stroke study. *Neurology* 2000; 55: 1649–1655.
7. Hacke W, Kaste M, Bluhmki E, *et al.*; ECASS Investigators. Thrombolysis with alteplase 3 to 4.5 hours after acute ischemic stroke. *N Engl J Med* 2008; 359: 1317–1329.
8. Mutzenbach JS, Pikija S, Otto F, *et al.* Intravenous thrombolysis in acute ischemic stroke after dabigatran reversal with idarucizumab: a case report. *Ann Clin Transl Neurol* 2016; 3: 889–892.

9. Khatri P, Kleindorfer DO, Devlin T, *et al.*; PRISMS Investigators. Effect of alteplase vs aspirin on functional outcome for patients with acute ischemic stroke and minor nondisabling neurologic deficits: the PRISMS randomized clinical trial. *JAMA* 2018; 320: 156–166.

10. Urrutia VC, Faigle R, Zeiler SR, *et al.* Safety of intravenous alteplase within 4.5 hours for patients awakening with stroke symptoms. *PLoS One* 2018; 13(5): e0197714.

11. Thomalla G, Simonsen CZ, Boutitie F, *et al.*; WAKE-UP Investigators. MRI-guided thrombolysis for stroke with unknown time of onset. *N Engl J Med* 2018; 379: 611–622.

12. Ma H, Campbell BCV, Parsons MW, *et al.*; EXTEND Investigators. Thrombolysis guided by perfusion imaging up to 9 hours after onset of stroke. *N Engl J Med* 2019; 380: 1795–1803. doi:10.1056/NEJMoa1813046.

13. Schwamm LH, Wu O, Song SS, *et al.*; MR WITNESS Investigators. Intravenous thrombolysis in unwitnessed stroke onset: MR WITNESS trial results. *Ann Neurol* 2018; 83: 980–993.

14. Davis SM, Donnan GA, Parsons MW, *et al.*; EPITHET investigators. Effects of alteplase beyond 3 h after stroke in the Echoplanar Imaging Thrombolytic Evaluation Trial (EPITHET): a placebo-controlled randomised trial. *Lancet Neurol* 2008; 7: 299–309.

15. Lansberg MG, Straka M, Kemp S, *et al.*; DEFUSE 2 study investigators. MRI profile and response to endovascular reperfusion after stroke (DEFUSE 2): a prospective cohort study. *Lancet Neurol* 2012; 11: 860–867.

16. Anderson CS, Robinson T, Lindley RI, *et al.*; ENCHANTED Investigators and Coordinators. Low-dose versus standard-dose intravenous alteplase in acute ischemic stroke. *N Engl J Med* 2016; 374: 2313–2323.

17. Logallo N, Novotny V, Assmus J, *et al.* Tenecteplase versus alteplase for management of acute ischaemic stroke (NOR-TEST): a phase 3, randomised, open-label, blinded endpoint trial. *Lancet Neurol* 2017; 16: 781–788.

18. Campbell BCV, Mitchell PJ, Churilov L, *et al.*; EXTEND-IA TNK Investigators. Tenecteplase versus alteplase before thrombectomy for ischemic stroke. *N Engl J Med* 2018; 378: 1573–1582.

19. Hill MD, Lye T, Moss H, *et al.* Hemi-orolingual angioedema and ACE inhibition after alteplase treatment of stroke. *Neurology* 2003; 60: 1525–1527.

20. NINDS t-PA Stroke Study Group. Generalized efficacy of t-PA for acute stroke: subgroup analysis of the NINDS t-PA Stroke Trial. *Stroke* 1997; 28: 2119–2125.

21. Patel SC, Levine SR, Tilley BC, *et al.*; National Institute of Neurological Disorders and Stroke rt-PA Stroke Study Group. Lack of clinical significance of early ischemic changes on computed tomography in acute stroke. *JAMA* 2001; 286: 2830–2838.

6

Endovascular Therapy

When used alone, intravenous and intra-arterial thrombolysis have yielded low recanalization rates of proximal large-vessel occlusions (LVO). The endovascular trials utilizing first-generation devices such as the Merci retriever and the Penumbra aspiration system were essentially neutral and failed to demonstrate superiority of mechanical thrombectomy over IV tPA (MR RESCUE, SYNTHESIS, IMS-III).[1-3] In 2015, however, six trials – MR CLEAN, EXTEND-IA, SWIFT PRIME, ESCAPE, REVASCAT, and THRACE – led to a fundamental shift in how we acutely manage LVOs today.[4-9] All six trials compared endovascular thrombectomy (EVT) to IV tPA alone and demonstrated clear superiority of thrombectomy in patients presenting within 6 hours from the time they were last known well (LKW) if they met specific imaging criteria. In addition to faster recanalization times and selection of patients with favorable imaging profiles, the long-awaited success of mechanical thrombectomy was in part made possible by the safer profile and higher recanalization rates offered by the newer clot retrieval devices known as stent retrievers or "stentrievers."

More recently, two large multicenter trials – DAWN and DEFUSE 3 – extended the time window for the use of mechanical thrombectomy in patients with LVOs to up to 24 hours from LKW, if they again met specific imaging criteria.[10,11] Wake-up strokes and strokes with "delayed" presentation will be discussed later in this chapter.

It is the responsibility of the practitioner in charge of the initial evaluation of the case to identify those patients eligible for EVT and activate the chain of actions that will lead to expedited clot retrieval. Planning a thrombectomy requires coordination between various teams including EMS, emergency medicine, vascular neurology, neurointerventionist, anesthesia, and neurointensive care teams.

■ Time is Still Important

While the "time window" for EVT is longer than for tPA, getting the artery open as fast as possible is equally important to achieve the best possible outcome. It has been estimated that every hour's delay in achieving recanalization by EVT results in 8% decreased probability of good outcome.[12] Each minute saved in onset-to-treatment time grants on average 4.2 days of extra healthy life, and every 20 minutes decrease in treatment delay leads to an average gain equivalent of 3 months of disability-free life.[13] Furthermore, in the delayed time window, as time elapses since symptom onset, the ability of collateral flow to sustain tissue viability gradually diminishes, and consequently fewer patients will have a favorable imaging profile and the amount of salvageable tissue is reduced.

■ Planning an Endovascular Case

Your patient is suspected or confirmed to have an LVO. Whether the patient is in your ED or being transferred from another facility, deciding to send a patient to the angiography suite for mechanical thrombectomy requires moving down the following sequence of steps in an expedited fashion:

1. Ensure patient receives intravenous thrombolysis if they qualify.
2. Review patient's eligibility for EVT.

3. Promptly discuss the case with the attending neurologist (or vascular neurologist if available), neurointerventionist, and neurointensivist.
4. Initiate transfer of the patient to the EVT center or, if already on site, facilitate transport to the interventional suite.
5. Obtain consent for the procedure.
6. Activate the interventional and anesthesia teams (this task can be carried by the interventional team as well).
7. Reassess patient eligibility for EVT if time has elapsed since the initial evaluation.

Each step is discussed in more detail below.

1. IS MY PATIENT ELIGIBLE TO RECEIVE IV tPA?

All patients presenting to the ED or requiring transfer to an EVT center should promptly receive tPA within the 3–4.5-hour window if they qualify. Waiting to see whether tPA has an effect before considering the patient for EVT is not recommended. Sometimes, because of an absolute contraindication to thrombolysis, such as presence of coagulopathy, active bleeding, a history of ICH, or being outside the time window, tPA will be omitted and the patient taken directly to EVT. The question whether tPA can be omitted in all patients going for EVT is being addressed in ongoing randomized studies. Existing data are inconclusive. For now, omitting tPA should only be considered in tPA-ineligible patients and perhaps in selected patients in whom the EVT procedure can be done very quickly after arrival at the ED.

2. IS MY PATIENT ELIGIBLE TO RECEIVE EVT?

a. **Age ≥ 18** – None of the available RCTs enrolled patients under 18 years of age. Some case reports and case series have however demonstrated high recanalization rates in patients < 18 years old.

b. **Favorable premorbid condition (mRS 0–1)** – In general, the recent
   trials required patients to have a good premorbid function (mRS 0 or 1)
   to be eligible for EVT. In our practice, however, we still do consider
   patients with baseline mRS 2–4 for EVT after discussion with family and
   assessment of possible gains from the patient's baseline condition. The
   amount of benefit to be expected in disabled patients is deserving of
   further study.

c. **Demonstrable LVO in ICA or MCA M1**
   - Whenever possible, patients should undergo a non-invasive
     angiographic study, such as a CTA, to confirm an LVO. In the case of
     CTA, this entails availability of the imaging modality, appropriate
     vascular access, and absence of contraindications to iodinated
     contrast (advanced renal failure or severe contrast allergy such as
     anaphylaxis). MRA is an alternative to CTA if the latter is not feasible.
     In some cases, the clinical picture is highly suggestive of an LVO and
     the angiographic study can reasonably be bypassed to get the patient
     to the interventional suite as fast as possible.
   - Most of the occlusions treated with EVT in the trials were in the
     distal ICA or proximal MCA M1. Occlusions of other vessels (MCA
     M2, MCA M3, ACA, PCA, basilar or vertebral arteries) were either
     excluded or underrepresented, so no strong evidence exists yet to
     claim benefit of EVT in those cases. Treatment of patients with
     relatively distal occlusions should be individualized, taking into
     consideration the severity of the deficit and difficulty accessing the
     clot. Patients with proximal carotid occlusive disease or dissection
     were also underrepresented in the randomized trials. While at
     relatively higher risk of procedural complications, these proximal
     lesions can be carefully negotiated to achieve successful distal
     thrombectomy. Whether the proximal lesions should be stented or
     have angioplasty at the time of thrombectomy will depend on
     anatomy, ability to access the distal clot, and adequacy of
     collaterals.

d. **Significant acute neurological deficits (NIHSS ≥ 6)** – Although some of the trials enrolled patients with lower NIHSS on presentation, there are insufficient data to document the benefit of EVT in that patient population. Further RCTs are required to study EVT in patients with minor, yet disabling, strokes and LVO.

e. **Favorable neuroradiographic findings** – Safe and efficacious clot retrieval depends on the absence of extensive ischemic changes (i.e., small infarct volumes) and the presence of a relatively large penumbra to salvage. A robust collateral circulation gives patients the ability to be considered for delayed reperfusion attempts. This becomes very important for patients presenting with wake-up strokes or strokes of delayed presentation (> 6 hours from LKW). The role of perfusion studies in the "early" window (up to 6 hours) is not very well established. In the "late" window (6–24 hours), however, these studies are important for the appropriate selection of patients for EVT.

- **Strokes presenting within 6 hours from LKW** – This section is based on the results of the following trials: MR CLEAN, EXTEND-IA, SWIFT PRIME, ESCAPE, REVASCAT, and THRACE (Table 6.1).

  i. **ASPECTS ≥ 6** – The ASPECTS scoring system is a tool to quickly and reliably obtain an estimate of the extent of ischemic changes. The majority of the 2015 trials used ASPECTS to select patients for EVT. ASPECTS ≥ 6 was associated with better outcome from EVT, whereas a score < 6 was associated with no benefit and potentially greater harm from reperfusion injury. The 2018 AHA/ASA guidelines for the early management of acute ischemic stroke give the estimation of ASPECTS a strong recommendation.[14]

  ii. **Small infarct core volumes and large penumbra–core mismatch** – SWIFT PRIME and EXTEND-IA showed benefit for patients with a small infarct core size (< 50 mL and < 70 mL, respectively), and a large mismatch ratio (> 1.8 and > 1.2, respectively). These studies used CT or MR perfusion coupled with

Table 6.1 Specific design characteristics and outcomes of the early-window interventional trials: MR CLEAN, ESCAPE, SWIFT PRIME, EXTEND-IA, and REVASCAT

Trial	Selection characteristics and outcomes
MR CLEAN	Less strict mRS and NIHSS inclusion criteria
	Did not select based on any specific radiographic criteria
	Lowest recanalization rate of all the studies (used IA tPA and first-generation devices in minority)
	Lowest effect size (NNT = 7)
ESCAPE	Used multiphase CTA
	Selected moderate-to-good collateral circulation filling (i.e., > 50% of MCA pial arterial circulation)
SWIFT PRIME	Used perfusion studies (MRI/CT) – core infarct and penumbra criteria
EXTEND-IA	Largest effect size (NNT = 3–4)
	Highest recanalization rate of all the studies
REVASCAT	Used CT or MRI ASPECTS

an automated software that calculates volumes and ratios based on designated CBF and T_{max} thresholds. However, the latest guidelines do not routinely recommend obtaining perfusion studies to determine patient eligibility for EVT in the early reperfusion window.

iii. **Collateral status** – ESCAPE further selected patients on the basis of collateral circulation. This study enrolled patients with moderate-to-good collaterals, defined as 50% or greater filling of MCA pial arterial circulation as seen on multiphase CTA.

- **Strokes presenting within 6–24 hours from LKW** – The DAWN and DEFUSE 3 trials addressed the topic of strokes with delayed presentation (Tables 6.2 and 6.3). DAWN enrolled patients 6–24 hours from LKW, while DEFUSE 3 limited the time window to 6–16 hours. The common feature between these two trials was the selection of patients on the basis of their infarct core–penumbra mismatch as obtained by

Table 6.2 Comparison of patient groups selected for mechanical thrombectomy in the extended time window in the DAWN and DEFUSE 3 trials

Clinical deficit–infarct volume mismatch (DAWN trial)	Infarct core–penumbra mismatch (DEFUSE 3 trial)
Group A: ≥ 80 y.o., NIHSS ≥ 10, infarct volume < 21 mL	Initial infarct volume < 70 mL
Group B: < 80 y.o., NIHSS ≥ 10, infarct volume < 31 mL	Mismatch ratio > 1.8
Group C: < 80 y.o., NIHSS ≥ 20, infarct volume 31–51 mL	

CT or MR perfusion studies and measured by automated software. In both trials, the infarct core was determined as the tissue with a CBF falling below 30% of the unaffected contralateral hemispheric CBF.

  i. **DAWN** – DAWN's particularity is that it looked at a clinical-radiographic mismatch. It categorized patients into three groups as depicted in Table 6.2. Patients in groups A and B had a statistically larger benefit from EVT compared to IV tPA alone.

 ii. **DEFUSE 3** – To be enrolled, patients had to have an initial infarct volume smaller than 70 mL and a penumbra–core mismatch ratio greater than 1.8. The penumbra was determined as the tissue with T_{max} longer than 6 seconds.

3. THREE-WAY DISCUSSION BETWEEN STROKE, NEUROINTERVENTIONIST, AND NEUROCRITICAL CARE TEAMS

a. Decision to go for mechanical thrombectomy requires the involvement of the vascular neurology, neurointerventionist, and neurocritical care teams.

Table 6.3 Comparison of DAWN and DEFUSE 3 trial selection characteristics and outcomes

Characteristics	DAWN	DEFUSE 3
Selection criteria		
Last known well (hours)	6–24	6–16
Age (years)	≥ 18	18–90
National Institute of Health Stroke scale	≥ 10	≥ 6
Baseline modified Rankin scale	0–1	0–2
Maximum infarct volume (mL)	51	70
Results		
Functional independence (modified Rankin scale 0–2, EVT vs. MM) at 90 days	49% vs. 13% ($p > 0.999$)	44.6% vs. 16.7% ($p < 0.001$)
Symptomatic ICH, EVT vs. MM	6% vs. 3% (non-significant)	7% vs. 4% (non-significant)
All-cause mortality, EVT vs. MM	19% vs. 18% (non-significant)	14% vs. 26% ($p = 0.05$)

EVT, endovascular therapy; MM, medical management; ICH, intracranial hemorrhage.

Source: Sheinberg DL, McCarthy DJ, Peterson EC, Starke RM. DEFUSE-3 Trial: reinforcing evidence for extended endovascular intervention time window for ischemic stroke. *World Neurosurg* 2018; 112: 275–276.[15] Reproduced with permission from Elsevier.

b. Once you have identified that (or are unsure whether) a patient is suitable for EVT, you should contact the attending neurologist or vascular neurologist on call and discuss the case with them. Ensuring that you have a maximum of pertinent information such as time of LKW, premorbid condition, labs, imaging, and neurological exam (NIHSS) will expedite the process and avoid delays.

c. Familiarity with how to contact the neurointerventionist team is also very helpful (pager numbers, on-call schedule, etc.).

d. After the procedure is completed, the patient will be admitted to the neurointensive care unit for close monitoring, creating the need to contact the ICU staff and keep them updated with the progress of the case. The ICU should be made aware of the patient upfront so that arrangements for bed assignment and personnel mobilization can be made.

4. FACILITATE TIMELY TRANSFER OF THE PATIENT TO THE INTERVENTIONAL SUITE

The patient could be in the emergency room, at an outside hospital, or in a different unit/floor within the hospital. Regardless of the location, it is the responsibility of the practitioner initially evaluating the patient to facilitate transfer to the angio suite.

This may mean physically helping with patient transport, or contacting the admitting office, bed management office, and/or air medical service your hospital is contracted with (if the patient is to be flown in).

5. OBTAIN CONSENT FOR THE PROCEDURE

Consent can be obtained from patient or family, or, if that is not possible, an emergency two-physician consent can be signed.

6. SHOULD MY PATIENT BE UNDER GENERAL ANESTHESIA OR CONSCIOUS SEDATION FOR THE PROCEDURE?

Until recently, retrospective studies had highlighted the concerns of intraprocedural hypotension with general anesthesia (GA), swaying the pendulum towards the use of conscious sedation (CS) for thrombectomy. However, three recently published RCTs – SIESTA, AnStroke, and GOLIATH – showed that GA was not inferior to CS.[16–18] Despite faster door-to-groin puncture time for CS (~10 minutes in SIESTA), there was no difference in early neurological deterioration at 24 hours and no difference in infarct volume. The GA group also tended to have better clinical outcomes at 90 days. The rate of procedural hypotensive episodes was very low and did not vary across the two groups, likely due to the utilization of expert neuroanesthesia care.

The main advantage of GA is reduced patient movement, whereas CS benefits from the possibility to get a neurological assessment during and immediately after the procedure. Disadvantages for GA include ventilation-related complications (e.g., delayed extubation, pneumothorax, pneumonia) and hypotensive episodes. On the other hand, CS may need to be emergently converted to GA during the procedure, which adds delay and complications.

The decision to proceed with GA or CS for thrombectomy must therefore be individualized, taking into consideration the patient's clinical status and the institution's resources and capabilities (e.g., presence of neuroanesthesia and neurocritical care services).

7. HAS SIGNIFICANT TIME ELAPSED BETWEEN THE DECISION TO TREAT AND THE INTERVENTION?

In the event the patient is nearing the end of the therapeutic time window, because of either late initial presentation or delayed transfer, we recommend a non-contrast head CT be performed to re-evaluate the extent of the ischemic burden (e.g., ASPECTS scoring), especially if further neurological deterioration has happened. This should, however, by no means add to the delay in getting the patient to the interventional suite.

■ During the Procedure

1. **Recanalization grading system**

   a. The goal of mechanical thrombectomy is reperfusion, which happens through recanalization of the occluded vessel and restoration of distal blood flow. Higher recanalization rates have strongly been associated with improved functional outcomes in the more recent EVT trials.

   b. We use the modified Thrombolysis in Cerebral Infarction (mTICI) grading system to assess extent and quality of recanalization (Table 6.4).

   c. We aim at achieving a grade of mTICI 2b or 3. This, sometimes, is unfortunately not feasible despite several passes of the stent retrievers and the use of adjuvant pharmacological agents such as intra-arterial tPA or heparin.

Table 6.4 Modified Thrombolysis in Cerebral Infarction (mTICI) angiographic response scale

mTICI score	Description
0	No perfusion
1	Perfusion past the initial occlusion, but limited distal branch filling with little or slow distal reperfusion
2a	Antegrade reperfusion of less than half of the previously occluded target-artery ischemic territory
2b	Antegrade reperfusion of more than half of the previously occluded target-artery ischemic territory
3	Complete antegrade reperfusion of the previously occluded target-artery ischemic territory, with absence of visualized occlusion in all distal branches

Adapted from: Zadat O, Yoo A, Khatri P, *et al.* Recommendations on angiographic revascularization grading standards for acute ischemic stroke: a consensus statement. *Stroke* 2013; 44: 2650–2663.[19]

2. **New devices improve success and safety of recanalization** – The newer stent retrievers have been associated with greater recanalization rates, improved functional outcomes, and an equal or better safety profile. In a single-center experience, stent retrievers achieved mTICI 2b/3 recanalization grade in 97% versus 80%, and good functional outcome (mRS ≤ 2) in 62% versus 23% cases compared with non-stent-retriever devices.[20] Stent retrievers have mostly replaced the earlier devices such as the Merci retriever. The Penumbra aspiration device is still used in selected cases. The stent retrievers deploy a stent across the thrombus, encaging it and then slowly retracting it into the guide catheter, through which suction is applied to reduce the risk of embolization. In some systems, a balloon is inflated proximally at the time of retraction to occlude blood flow so as to facilitate the retraction process. Currently, the two FDA-approved stent retrievers are the Solitaire FR and the Trevo, which mostly differ from one another by the enhanced visibility of the Trevo stent under fluoroscopy.

3. **Tandem occlusions**

   a. At times, there may be a more proximal cervical ICA stenosis (secondary to atherosclerosis or dissection) in addition to an intracranial occlusion. Even though the intracranial occlusion is usually the symptomatic lesion, the more proximal ICA stenosis can be significantly flow-limiting if not treated.

   b. While the approach differs among interventionists, if the thrombectomy device can be negotiated past the proximal carotid lesion which is not causing hemodynamic symptoms, the proximal lesion can be left alone. However, often it is necessary to address the cervical lesion before the intracranial clot can be removed, by either placing a stent or performing balloon angioplasty across the stenosis. Another reason would be if collateral circulation is poor and the proximal lesion is causing hemodynamic compromise.

    c. Placement of a carotid stent will require the use of dual antiplatelets (such as aspirin and clopidogrel) for at least 3 months to prevent in-stent thrombosis.

4. **Intraprocedural blood-pressure control** – If and when significant recanalization is achieved during the case, any sudden increase in blood pressure should be avoided to limit the risk of reperfusion injury. If SBP is ≤ 140, it is usually not necessary to lower the BP further. Any BP reduction should be done cautiously, so as not to induce hypoperfusion, especially in the case of residual clot burden. Dropping the BP too aggressively in this instance may worsen the deficits and expand the infarct zone. In one study, every 10 mmHg drop in mean arterial pressure (MAP) below 100 mmHg had an odds ratio (OR) of 1.28 for poor neurological outcome.[21] The 2018 AHA/ASA guidelines for the early management of acute ischemic stroke state that it may be reasonable to maintain BP < 180/105 mmHg during and for 24 hours after the procedure.[14] More data are needed to recommend more specific guidelines for BP control post-thrombectomy.

■ After the Procedure

1. **Need for initial ICU monitoring** – Post-procedure, the patient should be monitored in the ICU for at least 24 hours. During this time, blood pressure can be regulated as needed, any sign of deterioration can be promptly detected, and potential for development of malignant edema (and thus need for decompressive hemicraniectomy) can be assessed. In the ICU, the patient will receive neuro checks every 1–2 hours initially, with the plan of spacing them out as the patient's condition stabilizes.

2. **Antithrombotic use** – The use of antithrombotics will be determined by whether IV tPA was used, a stent was placed, or recanalization was not achieved leaving a worrisome high-grade stenosis.

a. If the patient received IV tPA, provided no stent was placed, we will wait for 24 hours and repeat a head CT, ensuring it is negative for hemorrhagic conversion before starting an antiplatelet agent.

b. If a stent was placed, the patient will need to be started right away on an antiplatelet (usually both aspirin and clopidogrel) because of the high risk of in-stent thrombosis. Antiplatelet loading (e.g., 300–600 mg of clopidogrel) is controversial and not universally done for stent placement.

c. If the procedure was not successful in opening up a tight intracranial stenosis which threatens to close at any time, or if there is residual intraluminal thrombus, an unproven approach is to infuse an antithrombotic agent for 12–24 hours in an attempt to prevent platelet aggregation and further thrombus formation. Examples of these agents include argatroban, abciximab, and heparin. This should be carefully discussed between the three teams participating in the patient's care.

3. **Care of the sheath or closure device**

a. The patient will need to remain flat with the leg that has had a groin puncture kept straight for a few hours. The length of immobilization depends on whether the sheath is still present or if a closure device was used.

b. If the sheath is still present (for quicker vascular re-access if needed), the leg will have to remain straight for 6–8 hours after the sheath is removed. The heparin infusing through the sheath will have to be stopped about 30 minutes before its removal. Direct pressure on the insertion site will have to be maintained for 10–20 minutes, or longer in the case of active bleeding.

c. If a closure device is used at the end of the procedure, then the duration of leg immobilization is shorter (2–4 hours).

d. The interventional team will typically be responsible for removal of the sheath.

4. **Serial distal pulses checks**

   a. Make sure there is no developing hematoma or pseudoaneurysm at the groin puncture site. Evidence of acute hemoglobin drop without another identifiable cause should prompt you to look for a retroperitoneal hemorrhage with a non-contrast CT of the abdomen and pelvis. Further dedicated vascular imaging and a vascular surgery consult may be warranted if the bleeding does not stop. Further management of iatrogenic retroperitoneal hemorrhage is beyond the scope of this text.

   b. Check distal pulses (posterior tibialis, dorsalis pedis) by palpation (or Doppler) and compare the two sides. If a pulse is not present and the limb is cold, this is a vascular emergency and vascular surgery should be immediately consulted.

■ Risks and Benefits of EVT

WHAT ARE THE BENEFITS OF EVT IN THE EARLY REPERFUSION WINDOW?

In HERMES, a meta-analysis pooling the data from five of the RCTs discussed above, the following conclusions were reached:[22]

1. There was significant improvement in functional independence at 90 days (mRS 0–2) for patients who underwent EVT compared to those who had standard of care with IV thrombolysis (IVT). The odds ratio (OR) was 2.39 (95% CI 1.88–3.04) (Figure 6.1).

2. There was no statistical difference in the all-cause mortality rate at 90 days between EVT and IVT (OR 0.80, 95% CI 0.60–1.07).

3. The rate of symptomatic ICH (defined as any ICH coupled with a deterioration in NIHSS of 4 points or more) was also not different between the two treatment arms (OR 1.11, 95% CI 0.66–1.87).

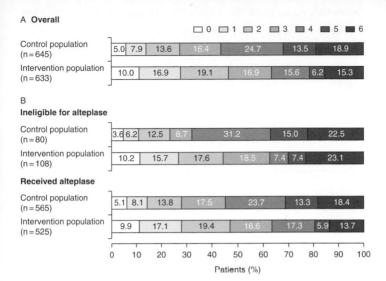

Figure 6.1 Functional outcome at 90 days as depicted by the modified Rankin scale (mRS) score distribution in endovascular therapy compared with medical management. (A black and white version of this figure will appear in some formats. For the color version, please refer to the plate section.)

Source: Goyal M, Menon BK, van Zwam WH, *et al.*; HERMES collaborators. Endovascular thrombectomy after large-vessel ischaemic stroke: a meta-analysis of individual patient data from five randomised trials. *Lancet* 2016; 387: 1723–1731.[22] Reproduced with permission.

4. The number needed to treat (NNT) to achieve functional independence at 90 days (mRS 0–2) with EVT compared to IV tPA alone was 5.26.

WHAT ARE THE BENEFITS OF EVT IN THE LATE REPERFUSION WINDOW?

1. Functional independence at 90 days was achieved in 49% for the EVT arm versus 13% for the standard-treatment arm in DAWN (NNT= 2.78)

and 44.6% versus 16.7% (NNT = 3.58) in DEFUSE 3. This large effect size is in part due to the radiographic selection of patients with slow-growing infarcts, but also due to the low performance of the control group, in which most patients were ineligible to receive tPA.

2. Again, there was no statistical difference in all-cause mortality or rate of symptomatic ICH between intervention and standard therapy in the two trials.

WHAT ARE THE RISKS OF EVT?

Reperfusion Risk

1. Recanalizing a vessel via thrombolysis or thrombectomy is associated with a risk of reperfusion injury, which manifests as hemorrhagic transformation and/or significant edema in the ischemic territory. This is more prevalent in tissues that are exposed to high perfusion pressures, those that are reperfused late, and those with poor collateral circulation.

2. In HERMES, the number needed to harm (NNH) for any ICH was 10, and that for symptomatic ICH was 517.

3. As mentioned above, avoiding hypertension after recanalization is a very important measure to prevent reperfusion injury. It is less clear by how much the blood pressure should be lowered.

Iatrogenic Complications

1. **Difficult vascular access** – Tortuous, thrombosed vessels or variant vascular anatomy can make thrombectomy very difficult, if not impossible at times. This is particularly true in patients with proximal carotid artery stenosis, dissection, or occlusion, and these patients were often excluded from the randomized trials. The preferred site for vascular access is the femoral artery, but if this approach is difficult or impossible, radial arteries can be used. The tortuosity of the vessels and, in some cases, the acute angle at which vessels take off from the

aorta can make delivery of the thrombectomy devices to the site of the clot very challenging.

2. **Distal showering of emboli** – This complication appears to be less common with the newer devices but occurred in ~5% of cases in the randomized trials. Distal protection devices are often deployed, but they can produce emboli themselves in the process of deployment.

3. **Vessel dissection** – This complication occurred in 4.5% with stent retrievers in a post hoc analysis of SWIFT PRIME, resulting in a 1.1% rate of symptomatic SAH.

4. **Groin complications** – The rate of complications caused by groin puncture (e.g., pseudoaneurysm at the puncture site, retroperitoneal hemorrhage, cold limb) was 7.9% with the use of a stent retriever in the same SWIFT PRIME post hoc analysis.

■ Posterior Circulation

Occlusions of the basilar, vertebral, and posterior cerebral arteries have been underrepresented in the various RCTs that have addressed the efficacy of mechanical thrombectomy. The main reasons are lower incidence rates of occlusions of the posterior circulation and the dismal outcome if acute basilar artery occlusions (BAO) are not recanalized. In the ENDOSTROKE registry, comprising 148 patients with BAO, 84% got EVT with stent retrievers, 79% were successfully recanalized, 34% patients had a mRS 0–2 at 3 months, and 35% died.[23]

Optimal timing of intervention in the posterior circulation is still unclear. Most interventions are carried out within 6 hours but some have been performed as late as 48 hours after symptom onset. The imaging profiles (low ASPECTS, small core, large mismatch) used for selecting anterior circulation stroke patients are not useful in the posterior circulation. However, similar to the anterior circulation, frank hypodensity on CT indicates non-salvageable tissue, so a very hypodense brainstem probably represents a futile situation. We often get an emergency MRI FLAIR sequence to assess brainstem viability in cases presenting beyond 6 hours from onset. Predictors of good outcomes following EVT are successful recanalization, low NIHSS score, and good collateral status. Successful recanalization is heavily dependent on thrombus length, clots shorter than 1 cm being associated with a 70–80% recanalization rate, as well as on clot location, distal being associated with more favorable outcomes than proximal occlusion sites.

BASICS, a multicenter RCT, is under way to compare the efficacy and safety of intra-arterial thrombolysis (with tPA or urokinase) compared to best medical management alone.[24] The use of stents is allowed in order to gain access to the BAO in case of vertebral artery stenosis/occlusion or if there is residual high-grade stenosis of the basilar artery after thrombolysis.

References

1. Kidwell CS, Jahan R, Gornbein J, *et al.*; MR RESCUE Investigators. A trial of imaging selection and endovascular treatment for ischemic stroke. *N Engl J Med* 2013; 368: 914–923.

2. Ciccone A, Valvassori L, Nichelatti M, *et al.*; SYNTHESIS Expansion Investigators. Endovascular treatment for acute ischemic stroke. *N Engl J Med* 2013; 368: 904–913.

3. Broderick JP, Palesch YY, Demchuk AM, *et al.*; Interventional Management of Stroke (IMS) III Investigators. Endovascular therapy after intravenous t-PA versus t-PA alone for stroke. *N Engl J Med* 2013; 368: 893–903.

4. Berkhemer OA, Fransen PS, Beumer D, *et al.*; MR CLEAN Investigators. A randomized trial of intraarterial treatment for acute ischemic stroke. *N Engl J Med* 2015; 372: 11–20.

5. Campbell BC, Mitchell PJ, Kleinig TJ, *et al.*; EXTEND-IA Investigators. Endovascular therapy for ischemic stroke with perfusion-imaging selection. *N Engl J Med* 2015; 372: 1009–1018.

6. Saver JL, Goyal M, Bonafe A, *et al.*; SWIFT PRIME Investigators. Stent-retriever thrombectomy after intravenous t-PA vs. t-PA alone in stroke. *N Engl J Med* 2015; 372: 2285–2295.

7. Goyal M, Demchuk AM, Menon BK, *et al.*; ESCAPE Trial Investigators. Randomized assessment of rapid endovascular treatment of ischemic stroke. *N Engl J Med* 2015; 372: 1019–1030.

8. Jovin TG, Chamorro A, Cobo E, *et al.*; REVASCAT Trial Investigators. Thrombectomy within 8 hours after symptom onset in ischemic stroke. *N Engl J Med* 2015; 372: 2296–2306.

9. Bracard S, Ducrocq X, Mas JL, *et al.*; THRACE investigators. Mechanical thrombectomy after intravenous alteplase versus alteplase alone after stroke (THRACE): a randomised controlled trial. *Lancet Neurol* 2016; 15: 1138–1147.

10. Nogueira RG, Jadhav AP, Haussen DC, *et al.*; DAWN Trial Investigators. Thrombectomy 6 to 24 hours after stroke with a mismatch between deficit and infarct. *N Engl J Med* 2018; 378: 11–21.

11. Albers GW, Marks MP, Kemp S, *et al.*; DEFUSE 3 Investigators. Thrombectomy for stroke at 6 to 16 hours with selection by perfusion imaging. *N Engl J Med* 2018; 378: 708–718.

12. Mulder MJHL, Jansen IGH, Goldhoorn RB, *et al.*; MR CLEAN Registry Investigators. Time to endovascular treatment and outcome in acute ischemic stroke: MR CLEAN registry results. *Circulation* 2018; 138: 232–240.

13. Meretoja A, Keshtkaran M, Tatlisumak T, Donnan GA, Churilov L. Endovascular therapy for ischemic stroke: save a minute–save a week. *Neurology* 2017; 88: 2123–2127.

14. Powers WJ, Rabinstein AA, Ackerson T, *et al.*; American Heart Association Stroke Council. 2018 guidelines for the early management of patients with acute ischemic stroke: a guideline for healthcare professionals from the American Heart Association/American Stroke Association. *Stroke* 2018; 49: e46–e110.

15. Sheinberg DL, McCarthy DJ, Peterson EC, Starke RM. DEFUSE-3 Trial: reinforcing evidence for extended endovascular intervention time window for ischemic stroke. *World Neurosurg* 2018; 112: 275–276.

16. Schönenberger S, Uhlmann L, Hacke W, *et al.* Effect of conscious sedation vs general anesthesia on early neurological improvement among patients with ischemic stroke undergoing endovascular thrombectomy: a randomized clinical trial. *JAMA* 2016; 316: 1986–1996.

17. Löwhagen Hendén P, Rentzos A, Karlsson JE, *et al.* General anesthesia versus conscious sedation for endovascular treatment of acute ischemic stroke: the AnStroke trial (Anesthesia During Stroke). *Stroke* 2017; 48: 1601–1607.

18. Simonsen CZ, Sørensen LH, Juul N, *et al.* Anesthetic strategy during endovascular therapy: general anesthesia or conscious sedation? (GOLIATH – General or Local

Anesthesia in Intra Arterial Therapy). A single-center randomized trial. *Int J Stroke* 2016; 11: 1045–1052.

19. Zadat O, Yoo A, Khatri P, *et al.* Recommendations on angiographic revascularization grading standards for acute ischemic stroke: a consensus statement. *Stroke* 2013; 44: 2650–2663.

20. Hentschel KA, Daou B, Chalouhi N, *et al.* Comparison of non-stent retriever and stent retriever mechanical thrombectomy devices for the endovascular treatment of acute ischemic stroke. *J Neurosurg* 2017; 126: 1123–1130.

21. Whalin MK, Halenda KM, Haussen DC, *et al.* Even small decreases in blood pressure during conscious sedation affect clinical outcome after stroke thrombectomy: an analysis of hemodynamic thresholds. *AJNR Am J Neuroradiol* 2017; 38: 294–298.

22. Goyal M, Menon BK, van Zwam WH, *et al.*; HERMES collaborators. Endovascular thrombectomy after large-vessel ischaemic stroke: a meta-analysis of individual patient data from five randomised trials. *Lancet* 2016; 387: 1723–1731.

23. Singer OC, Berkefeld J, Nolte CH, *et al.*; ENDOSTROKE Study Group. Mechanical recanalization in basilar artery occlusion: the ENDOSTROKE study. *Ann Neurol* 2015; 77: 415–424.

24. BASICS Study Group. The Basilar Artery International Cooperation Study (BASICS): study protocol for a randomised controlled trial. *Trials* 2013; 14: 200.

7

Neurological Deterioration in Acute Ischemic Stroke

Although, classically, stroke symptoms are maximal at onset and patients gradually recover over days, weeks, and months, patients sometimes deteriorate. People have termed the phenomenon stroke progression, stroke in evolution, stroke deterioration, and symptom fluctuation. There is no consistent terminology. The phenomenon occurs from different causes and is incompletely understood. Although the typical definition of a significant neurological deterioration in trials has been a gain of ≥ 1 point on item 1a (level of consciousness) or ≥ 4 points in the motor items of the NIHSS, any detectable deterioration should prompt careful assessment and a tailored work-up.

This chapter discusses the evaluation of potential causes, and approaches for treatment of each cause.

■ Probable Causes

1. Stroke enlargement (e.g., arterial stenosis or occlusion with worsening perfusion)
2. Drop in perfusion pressure
3. Recurrent stroke (not common)
4. Cerebral edema and mass effect
5. Hemorrhagic transformation

6. Metabolic disturbance (hypoxia, hypercarbia, decreased cardiac output, increased glucose, decreased sodium, fever, sedative drugs, etc.)
7. Seizure, post-ictal state
8. Symptom fluctuation without good cause (due to inflammation?)
9. The patient is not feeling like cooperating (sleepy, drugs)

■ Initial Evaluation of Patients with Neurological Deterioration

1. Check airway – breathing – circulation (ABC), vital signs, laboratory tests. Is the patient hypotensive or hypoxic?
2. Talk to and examine the patient. If the patient is sleepy, is it because it's 3 a.m. or because of mass effect? Is there a pattern of symptoms (global worsening versus focal worsening)?
3. Get an immediate non-contrast head CT (to evaluate for hemorrhage, new stroke, swelling, etc.).
4. Review medications (antihypertensives, sedatives).
5. Observe patient, and ask nurse, for subtle signs of seizure.
6. Consider MRI for brain imaging, new stroke, stroke enlargement, swelling; TCD or CT/MR angiography, CT/MR perfusion for arterial imaging; EEG to diagnose subclinical seizures. Chemistry, cultures, urinalysis, blood gases to rule out toxometabolic causes.
7. In some of these situations, the patient might benefit from closer monitoring in the neurointensive care unit.

■ Stroke Enlargement

This occurs when there is worsening or recurring arterial stenosis/occlusion and the hemodynamics change for some reason. There are no data to support that anticoagulation prevents hemodynamic worsening. The treatment should match what you think is the pathophysiology behind the deterioration.

Early treatment of the underlying stenosis/occlusion is undeniably the best course of action. The key is finding the high-risk patients early by performing imaging to detect large-artery stenosis/occlusion by CTA/MRA, TCD/carotid Doppler, or MRI. Patients with minor deficits but abnormal TCD, CTA, or MRA are at highest risk of progression. Perfusion imaging may indicate areas of tissue at risk. Even without an MR or CT perfusion study, the finding of a small diffusion-weighted lesion on MRI and a relatively minor neurological deficit in the presence of large-artery occlusion may indicate a high risk for progression. In such patients, you might want to consider early intervention, such as IV thrombolysis despite low NIHSS score, intra-arterial therapy, carotid endarterectomy, or carotid stenting.

Even if early treatment of the underlying stenosis/occlusion is not done, there are still treatment options for strokes that enlarge, especially in the current era of late-window reperfusion strategies (i.e., beyond 6 hours from LKW). Recent studies have shown that tPA may be effective if the FLAIR is not yet positive,[1] and thrombectomy improves outcome in patients with small ischemic core lesions up to 24 hours after stroke onset.[2,3] These data should be kept in mind and guide treatment when patients deteriorate on a hemodynamic basis after admission.

Reocclusion after thrombolysis/thrombectomy may also lead to substantial stroke enlargement. These patients may benefit from repeat angiography and thrombectomy if their imaging profile on perfusion studies is still favorable to intervention (see Chapter 6). The interventionist may repeat the thrombectomy and/or deploy a stent across a tight stenosis. If an intra-arterial thrombus is identified, heparin or a direct thrombin inhibitor drip (e.g., argatroban) should be considered.

Finally, if your deteriorating patient is not already on dual antiplatelets, this should be considered (see *Recurrent Stroke*, below).

■ Drop in Perfusion Pressure

Since autoregulation is compromised in ischemic brain, any reduction in blood pressure will reduce flow to penumbral regions, thereby potentially worsening the clinical deficit. This is true in both cortical and subcortical strokes. Lacunar strokes are notorious for fluctuating pressure-dependent symptoms due to the paucity of collateral flow in subcortical areas. As a rule of thumb, mean arterial pressure (MAP) should be kept at pre-stroke levels (as a general guideline, at least 130 mmHg in hypertensive patients, and 110 mmHg in normotensive patients) in the first 24 hours, and, if MAP drops below this level and the patient deteriorates, the MAP should be increased by fluid boluses and possibly initiation of a pressor. Some data suggest that blood-pressure fluctuations are particularly deleterious, so wide fluctuations in MAP should be avoided.

Laying patients flat may temporarily optimize cerebral perfusion and result in improvement in symptoms. The recent HeadPoST trial, which randomized patients to either lying flat or sitting up at 30 degrees for 24 hours post-stroke, showed no differences in stroke recovery at 90 days or rate of pneumonias.[4] However, this study mainly included patients with mild strokes, which may not have been the group most likely to benefit, and the intervention was not carried out in the first hours after stroke.

■ Recurrent Stroke

Unfortunately some patients go on to have recurrent strokes. Recent data suggest that most patients with acute non-cardioembolic strokes, and certainly those at highest risk of recurrent stroke such as those with intracranial atherosclerosis, multiple infarcts, or large-artery occlusion, should be treated with dual antiplatelets (aspirin + clopidogrel) starting within the first 24 hours (see Chapter 8).[5-7] Ticagrelor may be an alternative and is under study either alone or in combination with aspirin.

Among atrial fibrillation patients, the stroke recurrence risk is 5–8% in the first 2 weeks.[8-10] There are no data to show that immediate or "early" anticoagulation helps, even in the setting of atrial fibrillation, because anticoagulation can lead to hemorrhagic complications (see *Hemorrhagic Transformation*, below). Yet we might be underestimating the magnitude of frequency of stroke recurrence if we rely on clinical deterioration alone. One study reported that stroke recurrence was detected by MRI in 34% of patients in the first week, whereas clinically only 2% stroke recurrence was noted.[11] Furthermore, some patients may be at higher risk of re-embolization, especially those with associated mitral stenosis or left atrial thrombus. Therefore, our recommendation in atrial fibrillation patients is to anticoagulate once we determine by repeat brain imaging that the infarct is small or, if it is large, that any acute hemorrhagic transformation or vasogenic edema is resolving. This usually means waiting 48–96 hours after the acute stroke.

In a large population-based study, large-artery atherosclerosis was associated with the highest risk of stroke recurrence (Figure 7.1, Table 7.1).[12] This supports the recommendation to perform carotid revascularization (endarterectomy or stenting) earlier rather than later (see *Carotid Stenosis* in Chapter 8).

Table 7.1 Stroke mechanisms and risk of early recurrence

Mechanism	Recurrence at 1 week (95% CI)	Recurrence at 1 month (95% CI)	Recurrence at 3 months (95% CI)
Large-artery atherosclerosis (LAA)	4.0% (0.2–7.8)	12.6% (5.9–19.3)	19.2% (11.2–27.2)
Cardioembolism (CE)	2.5% (0.1–4.9)	4.6% (1.3–7.9)	11.9% (6.4–17.4)
Small-vessel stroke (SVS)	0%	2.0% (0–4.2)	3.4% (0.5–6.3)
Undetermined (UND)	2.3% (0.5–4.1)	6.5% (3.4–9.6)	9.3% (5.6–13.0)

Source: Lovett JK, Coull AJ, Rothwell PM. Early risk of recurrence by subtype of ischemic stroke in population-based incidence studies. *Neurology* 2004; 62: 569–573.[12] Reproduced with permission.

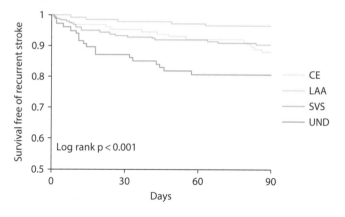

Figure 7.1 Stroke recurrence risk by stroke mechanism. (A black and white version of this figure will appear in some formats. For the color version, please refer to the plate section.) *Source:* Lovett JK, Coull AJ, Rothwell PM. Early risk of recurrence by subtype of ischemic stroke in population-based incidence studies. *Neurology* 2004; 62: 569–573.[12] Reproduced with permission.

■ Cerebral Edema and Mass Effect

This is a worry with large strokes, such as large MCA strokes involving the basal ganglia, often with some involvement of the ACA or PCA territories as well, and large cerebellar strokes. It is particularly concerning in young patients who do not have much atrophy and thus not much room for the brain to swell inside the skull. Monitor for any neurological change, decline in level of consciousness, rising blood pressure, periodic breathing, hiccups, headache, new cranial nerve abnormalities, and pupils (late phenomenon).

MEDICAL MANAGEMENT

1. Reduction of intracranial pressure (ICP) starts with head-of-bed positioning at > 30 degrees, head in neutral position to optimize venous outflow, immediate correction of fever, electrolyte imbalance, and hyperglycemia, and careful optimization of MAP and cardiac output to ensure adequate cerebral perfusion (cerebral perfusion pressure = MAP − ICP; should be kept ≥ 60 mmHg).

2. Osmotherapy (i.e., mannitol or hypertonics) is a temporizing measure that may help in some cases. Give mannitol (1–1.5 g/kg bolus over 30–60 minutes) upon signs of deterioration. The aim is to increase baseline serum osmolality by 10%, but no higher than 320 mOsm. Check serum osmolality every 12 hours and hold mannitol if > 320 mOsm. Hypertonics (e.g., 3% or 23.4% NaCl) can also be bolused to achieve the same effect. Intubation and mechanical ventilation (maintain SpO_2 > 95% and $PaCO_2$ 30–35 mmHg), judicious sedation, and at times paralysis may be necessary to control ICP.

3. Importantly, do not give steroids after a stroke (grade A recommendation). Randomized studies have shown that steroids may be more harmful than beneficial after an acute stroke.

SURGICAL THERAPY

1. Obtain a neurosurgical consultation early. For large MCA infarcts, consider early decompressive hemicraniectomy. The skull is taken off and a durotomy is made so that the brain can swell out rather than compress the brainstem (see below).

2. Pooled analyses from three European randomized controlled trials (DECIMAL, HAMLET, DESTINY) of patients under age 60 with malignant infarction in the MCA treated within 48 hours of stroke onset showed a statistically significant decrease in mortality and improvement in functional outcome with surgery (Figure 7.2).[13-15] At 1 year, there was a 50% absolute risk reduction of death, a 51% reduction in severe disability or death (mRS > 4), and a 23% absolute reduction in moderately severe disability or worse (mRS > 3).

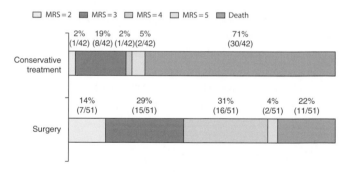

Figure 7.2 Pooled analysis comparing outcomes of decompressive hemicraniectomy and control groups among patients with malignant MCA stroke under the age of 60. (A black and white version of this figure will appear in some formats. For the color version, please refer to the plate section.)

Source: Vahedi K, Hofmeijer J, Juettler E, *et al.* Early decompressive surgery in malignant infarction of the middle cerebral artery: a pooled analysis of three randomised controlled trials. *Lancet Neurol* 2007; 6: 215–222.[16] Reproduced with permission.

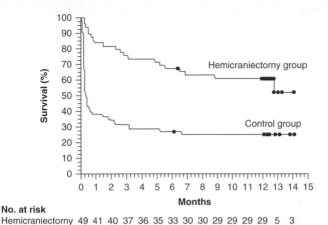

Figure 7.3 Kaplan–Meier survival curves comparing hemicraniectomy and control groups among patients over 60 years old with malignant MCA stroke.
Source: DESTINY II Investigators. Hemicraniectomy in older patients with extensive middle-cerebral-artery stroke. *N Engl J Med* 2014; 370: 1091–1100.[17] Reproduced with permission.

Number needed to treat (NNT) was 2 for survival avoiding severe disability and 4 for avoidance of moderately severe disability. Fourteen percent of individuals who underwent surgery achieved slight disability, being able to look after their own affairs without assistance (mRS 2).[16]

3. DESTINY II showed that patients > 60 years old who underwent decompressive hemicraniectomy within 48 hours of a malignant MCA infarct had greater survival but no improvement in functional independence (Figure 7.3).[17]

4. For cerebellar strokes, a ventriculostomy or external ventricular drain (EVD) is not sufficient as it may precipitate ascending transtentorial herniation. The appropriate treatment is suboccipital craniectomy ± EVD ± cerebellectomy.

5. With these procedures, a common error is restricting the size of the craniectomy, resulting in inadequate decompression. Landmarks for adequate craniectomy are included below as a guide, and Figure 7.4 shows an outline of the surgical method.

6. Of note, studies have not reported any difference in outcome between strokes involving the dominant (usually left hemisphere with significant aphasia) and non-dominant hemisphere. The side of such a large stroke should not influence the decision-making for hemicraniectomy.

CRITERIA FOR CONSIDERATION OF HEMICRANIECTOMY

- 5 hours from onset; > 50% MCA territory hypodense on CT
- 48 hours from onset; complete MCA territory hypodense on CT
- > 7.5 mm midline shift
- > 4 mm midline shift with lethargy
- Age < 60 years
- 145 mL infarct volume on MRI

Inclusion criteria from the pooled trials:

- Age 18–60 years
- Clinical deficits suggestive of infarction in the MCA with NIHSS > 15
- Altered LOC with a score of ≥ 1 on item 1a of the NIHSS
- Infarct of at least 50% of the MCA territory with or without additional infarction in the ipsilateral ACA or PCA territories on CT scan, or infarct volume > 145 mL on DWI sequence on MRI
- Inclusion within 45 hours after onset of symptoms

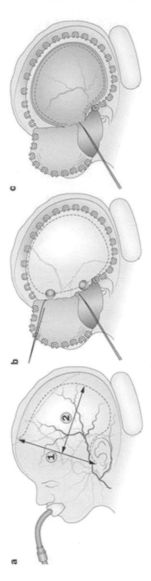

Figure 7.4 Technique for decompressive hemicraniectomy and durotomy. (A black and white version of this figure will appear in some formats. For the color version, please refer to the plate section.)

Source: Kolias AG, Kirkpatrick PJ, Hutchinson PJ. Decompressive craniectomy: past, present and future. *Nat Rev Neurol* 2013; 9: 405–415.[18] Reproduced with permission.

GUIDELINES FOR ADEQUATE SURGICAL DECOMPRESSION

The following landmarks and guidelines are derived from ongoing clinical trials:

- Anterior: frontal to mid-pupillary line
- Posterior: 4 cm posterior to external auditory canal
- Superior: superior sagittal sinus
- Inferior: floor of middle cranial fossa
- Durotomy over the entire region of decompression
- Dural grafting
- Other criteria include: 12 cm diameter craniectomy

■ Hemorrhagic Transformation

This should be clearly visible on non-contrast head CT (Figure 7.5; see also Figure 4.2). Most of the time, the patient is asymptomatic from the hemorrhagic transformation (also known as hemorrhagic conversion), unless it is large or in a critical location. Radiographically, hemorrhagic transformation is divided into four categories.[19]

- Hemorrhagic infarctions 1 and 2 (HI-1 and HI-2) represent petechial bleeding into the area of infarct without mass effect and are rarely symptomatic. HI-1 are small petechiae; HI-2 are confluent. If HI occurs, usually there is not much you can do or should do, except to stop antiplatelets and anticoagulants temporarily until you are sure there is no continued bleeding on repeat brain imaging.
- Parenchymal hemorrhages 1 and 2 (PH-1 and PH-2) represent confluent bleeding. If the bleeding takes up more than 30% of the infarcted area and produces mass effect (PH-2), it usually produces neurological deterioration. The risk of developing PH-2 is the main reason why anticoagulation is not recommended immediately after cardioembolic

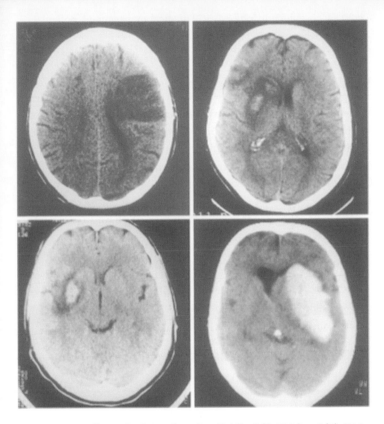

Figure 7.5 Types of hemorrhagic transformation: HI-1 (top left), HI-2 (top right), PH-1 (bottom left), and PH-2 (bottom right).
Source: Fiorelli M, Bastianello S, von Kummer R, *et al.* Hemorrhagic transformation within 36 hours of a cerebral infarct: relationships with early clinical deterioration and 3-month outcome in the European Cooperative Acute Stroke Study I (ECASS I) cohort. *Stroke* 1999; 30: 2280–2284.[19] Reproduced with permission.

stroke, and without repeat brain imaging first. PH should be managed similarly to any other cerebral hemorrhage: ABCs, blood-pressure control, coagulopathy reversal, ICP medical management, potential surgical decompression ± evacuation (Chapter 12).

■ Metabolic Disturbance

These are pretty self-explanatory. Remember that a sick brain is more sensitive to the effects of metabolic perturbations, so these should be sought and aggressively treated. In fact, such "post-stroke recrudescence" has gained greater attention as a very common explanation for a patient having worsening of pre-existing symptoms/signs.[20]

1. Mild fever or changes in sodium or glucose may have an exaggerated clinical effect.
2. Any intercurrent infection such as urinary tract infection or pneumonia will magnify the neurological findings.
3. Reduced cardiac output is a particularly bad comorbidity resulting in worse clinical outcome, and should be carefully avoided by optimizing fluid and inotropic therapy.
4. Remember also that "if the lips are blue, the brain is too," so look for, determine the cause of, and treat arterial oxygen desaturation. Possible causes:
   • pulmonary embolism
   • pneumonia
   • pulmonary edema
   • obstructive sleep apnea
5. Anemia: there is no widely accepted hemoglobin threshold for transfusion.
6. Sedative drugs interfere with rapid transition to rehabilitation mode and have also been associated with worse outcome, decreased mobilization with increased DVT risk, etc. Sedating drugs should be avoided as far as possible. See *The Uncooperative Patient*, below.

■ Seizure

Seizures occur in roughly 20% of all strokes, and are somewhat more frequent after hemorrhage than infarct. Most of the time, if seizures occur, they will appear at the time of stroke onset or within 24 hours. Seizures will often cause a post-ictal depressed level of consciousness, as well as worsening of the focal signs. Most authorities recommend withholding anticonvulsants unless the seizures are recurrent. Status epilepticus after acute stroke is exceedingly rare.

Intubation may be necessary to protect the airway in patients who already are impaired from their stroke. Aspiration pneumonia is common after seizures and should be assumed to occur if the seizure is generalized or intubation is necessary.

Newer anticonvulsants are being introduced, so current treatment guidelines should be consulted. The most common drugs used are:

- levetiracetam – 500 mg every 12 hours
- lamotrigine – 25 mg per day
- fosphenytoin – 20 mg/kg IV followed by maintenance phenytoin 200–300 mg per day
- valproate sodium – 10–15 mg/kg per day

■ Symptom Fluctuations Without a Good Cause

Some patients deteriorate without an obvious explanation.[21] This is a poorly understood phenomenon. It is commonly seen with subcortical strokes. While this usually occurs in the first 3 days, it can occur up to 2 weeks after stroke onset. The mechanism is unknown. Local blood–brain barrier disruption, hypoperfusion, inflammation, neurochemical or neurotransmitter changes, and apoptosis have all been posited but are unproven. Treatment is mainly supportive (maintain euvolemia, check blood pressure to make sure it does not drop). Anti-inflammatory (i.e., high-dose statins) and other neuroprotective therapies are under evaluation.

■ The Uncooperative Patient

Patients can become confused after a stroke. Contributing factors include advanced age and underlying dementia, placement in a disorienting critical-care environment, and sleep deprivation. Often, movement to a quiet private room helps, but this has to be balanced against less close scrutiny and treatment of medical complications outside the stroke unit or ICU setting. While sedation should be avoided, low doses of antipsychotic agents can be useful and are used commonly in case of agitation that may be harmful to the patient or to others – such as haloperidol PO or IV, risperidone PO, and quetiapine PO (see also *Delirium* in Chapter 15). There are also data to suggest that newer antipsychotic agents increase mortality of patients with dementia, though this was with prolonged treatment (10–12 weeks).[22] Therefore, pharmacologic management of agitation and confusion should be practiced with caution. Good nursing care, orientation, and calm environment are paramount.

References

1. Thomalla G, Simonsen CZ, Boutitie F, *et al.*; WAKE-UP Investigators. MRI-guided thrombolysis for stroke with unknown time of onset. *N Engl J Med* 2018; 379: 611–622.
2. Nogueira RG, Jadhav AP, Haussen DC, *et al.*; DAWN Trial Investigators. Thrombectomy 6 to 24 hours after stroke with a mismatch between deficit and infarct. *N Engl J Med* 2018; 378: 11–21.
3. Albers GW, Marks MP, Kemp S, *et al.*; DEFUSE 3 Investigators. Thrombectomy for stroke at 6 to 16 hours with selection by perfusion imaging. *N Engl J Med* 2018; 378: 708–718.

4. Anderson CS, Arima H, Lavados P, *et al.*; HeadPoST Investigators and Coordinators. Cluster-randomized, crossover trial of head positioning in acute stroke. *N Engl J Med* 2017; 376: 2437–2447.

5. Johnston SC, Easton JD, Farrant M, *et al.* Clopidogrel and aspirin in acute ischemic stroke and high-risk TIA. *N Engl J Med* 2018; 379: 215–225.

6. Wang Y, Wang Y, Zhao X, *et al.*; CHANCE Investigators. Clopidogrel with aspirin in acute minor stroke or transient ischemic attack. *N Engl J Med* 2013; 369: 11–19.

7. Chimowitz MI, Lynn MJ, Derdeyn CP, *et al.*; SAMMPRIS Trial Investigators. Stenting versus aggressive medical therapy for intracranial arterial stenosis. *N Engl J Med* 2011; 365: 993–1003.

8. Berge E, Abdelnoor M, Nakstad PH, Sandset PM. Low molecular-weight heparin versus aspirin in patients with acute ischaemic stroke and atrial fibrillation: a double-blind randomised study. HAEST Study Group. Heparin in Acute Embolic Stroke Trial. *Lancet* 2000; 355: 1205–1210.

9. Hart RG, Palacio S, Pearce LA. Atrial fibrillation, stroke, and acute antithrombotic therapy: analysis of randomized clinical trials. *Stroke* 2002; 33: 2722–2727.

10. Saxena R, Lewis S, Berge E, Sandercock PA, Koudstaal PJ. Risk of early death and recurrent stroke and effect of heparin in 3169 patients with acute ischemic stroke and atrial fibrillation in the International Stroke Trial. *Stroke* 2001; 32: 2333–2337.

11. Kang DW, Latour LL, Chalela JA, Dambrosia J, Warach S. Early ischemic lesion recurrence within a week after acute ischemic stroke. *Ann Neurol* 2003; 54: 66–74.

12. Lovett JK, Coull AJ, Rothwell PM. Early risk of recurrence by subtype of ischemic stroke in population-based incidence studies. *Neurology* 2004; 62: 569–573.

13. Vahedi K, Vicaut E, Mateo J, *et al.*; DECIMAL Investigators. Sequential-design, multicenter, randomized, controlled trial of early decompressive craniectomy in malignant middle cerebral artery infarction (DECIMAL Trial). *Stroke* 2007; 38: 2506–2517.

14. Hofmeijer J, Kappelle LJ, Algra A, *et al.*; HAMLET Investigators. Surgical decompression for space-occupying cerebral infarction (the Hemicraniectomy After Middle Cerebral Artery infarction with Life-threatening Edema Trial [HAMLET]): a multicentre, open, randomised trial. *Lancet Neurol* 2009; 8: 326–333.

15. Jüttler E, Schwab S, Schmiedek P, *et al.*; DESTINY Study Group. Decompressive Surgery for the Treatment of Malignant Infarction of the Middle Cerebral Artery (DESTINY): a randomized, controlled trial. *Stroke* 2007; 38: 2518–2525.

16. Vahedi K, Hofmeijer J, Juettler E, *et al.* Early decompressive surgery in malignant infarction of the middle cerebral artery: a pooled analysis of three randomised controlled trials. *Lancet Neurol* 2007; 6: 215–222.

17. Jüttler E, Unterberg A, Woitzik J, *et al.*; DESTINY II Investigators. Hemicraniectomy in older patients with extensive middle-cerebral-artery stroke. *N Engl J Med* 2014; 370: 1091–1100.

18. Kolias AG, Kirkpatrick PJ, Hutchinson PJ. Decompressive craniectomy: past, present and future. *Nat Rev Neurol* 2013; 9: 405–415.

19. Fiorelli M, Bastianello S, von Kummer R, *et al.* Hemorrhagic transformation within 36 hours of a cerebral infarct: relationships with early clinical deterioration and 3-month outcome in the European Cooperative Acute Stroke Study I (ECASS I) cohort. *Stroke* 1999; 30: 2280–2284.

20. Topcuoglu MA, Saka E, Silverman SB, *et al.* Recrudescence of deficits after stroke: clinical and imaging phenotype, triggers, and risk factors. *JAMA Neurol* 2017; 74: 1048–1055.

21. Vahidy FS, Hicks WJ, Acosta I, *et al.* Neurofluctuation in patients with subcortical stroke. *Neurology* 2014; 83: 398–405.

22. Schneider LS, Dagerman KS, Insel P. Risk of death with atypical antipsychotic drug treatment for dementia: meta-analysis of randomized placebo-controlled trials. *JAMA* 2005; 294: 1934–1943.

Ischemic Stroke Etiology and Secondary Prevention

In this chapter, we discuss mainly secondary prevention for stroke, although many of the measures, especially control of risk factors and lifestyle changes such as not smoking, controlling blood pressure, etc., are also important measures to avoid a first stroke.

Initially, we discuss a tailored diagnostic work-up, then general measures for secondary prevention of ischemic stroke, and finally recommendations for specific conditions that are associated with a high risk of recurrent stroke.

It is important to educate your patients and their families so they can take an active role in their health care and secondary stroke prevention. Also, as soon as possible, try to convert patients to the medications that they will be going home on prior to discharge, to make sure they tolerate them. Always take cost issues into account. A patient who cannot afford medications will not take them.

■ Diagnostic Studies

The goal of the "stroke work-up" is to find the cause of the stroke in order to determine the best treatment options to maximize the chance of preventing another stroke. There is no "cookbook" work-up for ischemic stroke. It is important to consider the patient's non-modifiable risk factors (age, sex), modifiable risk factors, and stroke syndrome when determining the extent of the diagnostic evaluation. For instance, a 75-year-old with longstanding hypertension, diabetes, and hypercholesterolemia and a lacunar infarct confirmed on brain imaging may need little additional work-up beyond a carotid ultrasound and ECG. However, a 40-year-old with no known risk factors and an acute stroke would require an extensive evaluation.

The following is a list of the studies that we consider in most stroke patients to distinguish stroke subtype and tailor our preventive measures. In Chapter 10, we will address the additional evaluation for young stroke patients with no risk factors, and others where the underlying cause may be more obscure.

In addition to the following, almost all stroke patients should have a complete blood count, electrolytes, creatinine, glucose, PT/PTT, electrocardiogram, and monitoring of heart rhythm by telemetry.

MRI OF THE BRAIN/MRA OF THE NECK AND BRAIN

- To localize the lesion.
- To try to understand the mechanism by integrating all MRI and MRA data:
  - small-vessel lacunar infarction
  - large-artery atherosclerosis
  - embolism
  - hemodynamic
  - venous
- The location and pattern of infarct(s) are helpful to determine etiology (watershed may refer to stenosis, whereas multiple vascular territories may suggest cardioembolic, etc.).
- To visualize what's acute using DWI and what's old using T2/FLAIR. Old strokes may help to determine etiology.

- To understand the tissue physiology (perfusion imaging).
- To examine the entire cervical and cerebral vasculature for stenosis (atherosclerosis, dissection, etc.), aneurysm, arteriovenous malformation (AVM).

REPEAT HEAD CT

Consider if patient is not able to have MRI.
- To localize the lesion.
- To look for hemorrhagic transformation of the infarct.
- To evaluate the deteriorating patient:
  - blood
  - cerebral edema
  - enlargement of infarct

CT ANGIOGRAM (CTA) OF THE NECK AND BRAIN

May be performed with the head CT in the acute evaluation, as an alternative to MRA.
- To look for extracranial or intracranial arterial stenosis, dissection, aneurysm.

TRANSTHORACIC ECHOCARDIOGRAM (TTE)

Order with "bubble study."
- To assess for embolic source (anterior wall or apical akinesis, clot, valvular disease, large PFO).
- Low ejection fraction (20–30% is generally agreed upon as a cutoff) significantly increases thromboembolic risk due to stasis, and also should trigger further specific cardiac evaluation and treatment. Left

atrial enlargement may signify valvular disease, occult atrial fibrillation, or atrial cardiopathy.

TRANSESOPHAGEAL ECHOCARDIOGRAM (TEE)

Order with "bubble study."
- To assess for embolic source not seen well on TTE (aortic atheroma, PFO, atrial septal aneurysm, spontaneous echo contrast, left atrial appendage clot).
- If a PFO is found, consider screening for hypercoagulable states, a bilateral lower-extremity ultrasound, and MR venogram of the pelvis to look for venous thrombosis. See discussion on *Patent Foramen Ovale* at the end of this chapter.

CAROTID ULTRASOUND (CUS)

- To assess for internal carotid artery stenosis or occlusion and direction of vertebral artery flow.
- You might not need it if you have a good-quality normal MRA or CTA of the extracranial circulation. CUS can be used to confirm a stenosis seen on MRA or CTA. If these non-invasive tests are concordant, it may not be necessary to do an invasive DSA to determine candidacy for endovascular or surgical treatment of a carotid stenosis.
- Also gives you a non-invasive benchmark for following carotid lesions longitudinally.
- CUS may also show high-risk ulcerated plaques, and can be used with transcranial Doppler (below) for emboli detection.

TRANSCRANIAL DOPPLER (TCD)

Order with or without "bubble study."
- To monitor clot presence and lysis in the acute setting.
- To confirm intracranial stenosis/occlusion of major arteries seen on MRA or CTA.
- To be used for emboli detection/monitoring.
- To screen for PFO by injecting microbubbles. TCD with "bubble study" is the most sensitive and least expensive/invasive way to screen for right-to-left shunting (whether intracardiac or intrapulmonary). See Appendix 2.
- To test hemodynamic reserve (breath-holding index [BHI], vasomotor reactivity).
- To evaluate collateral flow patterns.

DIGITAL SUBTRACTION ANGIOGRAPHY (DSA)

- Gold standard for determining degree of stenosis.
- Most sensitive way to definitively delineate and follow aneurysms or AVMs, dissection, vasculitis, or other arteriopathies.

FASTING LIPIDS

- Establish baseline for total cholesterol, triglycerides, LDL (target LDL < 70 mg/dL), HDL.

HEMOGLOBIN A1C (HGBA1C)

- Screen for diabetes and its recent control.

■ Control Risk Factors

1. BLOOD PRESSURE CONTROL

Hypertension is the single most important modifiable stroke risk factor. The risk of cardiovascular disease, beginning at BP 115/75 mmHg, doubles with each increment of 20/10 mmHg.[1] Multiple large randomized controlled trials (RCTs) have shown the efficacy of antihypertensive treatment in primary and secondary prevention of stroke. Many drugs have been shown to reduce stroke in primary prevention (beta-blocker in SHEP, diuretic in SHEP and ALLHAT, calcium channel blocker in ALLHAT, ACE inhibitor in HOPE and PROGRESS, ARB in LIFE).[2–6] A combination of perindopril (Aceon), a tissue-specific ACE inhibitor, and indapamide (Lozol), a diuretic, has been shown to reduce stroke in secondary prevention even among non-hypertensive patients (PROGRESS).[4] Whether this effect is due to the tissue-specific ACE inhibition rather than an ACE-inhibitor class effect, or whether an ACE inhibitor needs to be used in combination with a diuretic, remains unclear. Recent meta-analysis seems to support the superiority of diuretics.[7] The most important point is blood-pressure reduction, not the specific drug.

Guidelines for treatment of high blood pressure in adults were revised in 2017.[8] Treatment should begin with lifestyle modification including exercise, diet and salt restriction, and reduced alcohol. Pharmacologic treatment in patients with vascular disease including stroke should occur for SBP ≥ 140 or DBP ≥ 90. In general, bring down BP slowly with oral antihypertensives after acute ischemic stroke. A reduction of MAP by no more than 15% in the first 24 hours is reasonable, especially if there is large-vessel occlusive disease. Guidelines recommend starting with a thiazide diuretic as a first-line pharmacologic therapy, recognizing that more than one drug is commonly needed. In the hospital setting, especially after a stroke, a patient's fluid intake may be poor. A diuretic while on IV fluids does not make sense. Start a diuretic in stroke inpatients only if the patient is drinking fluids consistently. The usual first choice is an ACE inhibitor or calcium channel blocker. ACE inhibitors are less effective as monotherapy in African-Americans. If tachycardia is an issue, a beta-blocker can be useful, though not typically first line as a blood-pressure reducing agent.

In patients with severe hypertension, we usually start with IV nicardipine or labetalol to control the SBP to < 180 in patients after tPA, SBP ~140 in patients with acute ICH, and SBP 120–140 after successful endovascular revascularization. We transition to oral agents as soon as possible. We avoid the use of medications that require multiple daily dosing, because adherence to therapy is less likely if such agents are used.

According to recent guidelines, influenced by the SPRINT trial, the target BP for patients with atherosclerotic cardiovascular disease is ≤ 130/80 mmHg.[9] It is important to note that patients with stroke were excluded from this trial. However, based on prior studies in stroke patients, we agree that it is reasonable to target BP < 130/80 mmHg in patients with small-vessel ischemic stroke or intracerebral hemorrhage. In patients with extensive atherosclerotic disease and elderly patients, BP < 140/90 mmHg may be more practical. We expect that the stroke-specific secondary prevention guidelines will update blood-pressure recommendations for secondary stroke prevention.

2. LIPID CONTROL

The most recent American College of Cardiology (ACC) and American Heart Association (AHA) guidelines for the management of cholesterol revised their recommendations in patients with atherosclerotic cardiovascular disease (ASCVD), including those with ischemic stroke or transient ischemic attack (TIA).[10] These guidelines recommend initiation of high-dose statins (atorvastatin 40 or 80 mg or rosuvastatin 20 or 40 mg) for ASCVD regardless of the patient's age (in the past, this recommendation was only for patients < 75 years old).

The target of LDL < 70 mg/dL was influenced by the SPARCL trial. The SPARCL trial compared placebo with 80 mg of atorvastatin in patients with recent TIA/stroke with no known coronary artery disease or diabetes mellitus with LDL 100–190 mg/dL (2.6–4.9 mmol/L). LDL was lowered to < 70 mg/dL in the treatment group. Treatment with atorvastatin 80 mg was associated with a 2.2% 5-year absolute risk reduction (ARR) in fatal or non-fatal stroke and a 3.5% 5-year ARR in major cardiovascular events. There was a small increase in the incidence of hemorrhagic strokes.[11]

In order to assess patient adherence to therapy with statins and the effectiveness of statins at decreasing LDL cholesterol, we obtain a baseline lipid panel in the acute setting and a repeat lipid panel 8–12 weeks after statin initiation.

We recommend starting with a statin based on the ACC/AHA guidelines. If target LDL is not achieved, ezetimibe can be added, and if the target is still not reached, a PCSK-9 inhibitor.

Statins may benefit patients more than just by the amount they lower cholesterol. This mechanism is not entirely defined. The MRC/BHF Heart Protection Study treated patients with coronary artery disease or other occlusive arterial disease, or diabetes mellitus, with simvastatin or placebo irrespective of initial cholesterol concentrations and found significant reductions in MI, stroke, and revascularization procedures.[12]

3. HYPERGLYCEMIA AND INSULIN RESISTANCE

Guidelines state that hyperglycemia during the first 24 hours after acute ischemic stroke is associated with worse outcomes, and that it is reasonable to treat hyperglycemia to achieve blood glucose levels in the range of 140–180 mg/dL.[13] However, this is a class C recommendation.

A large randomized study recently showed that more aggressive glucose lowering (to 80–130 mg/dL) did not result in better 3-month outcome than more relaxed treatment (to 140–180 mg/dL).[14]

Diabetic patients should have appropriate education, diet counseling, and pharmacotherapy started before discharge.

Insulin resistance may be a target for secondary stroke prevention. Insulin resistance can be defined by the homeostasis model assessment of insulin resistance (HOMA-IR) index (fasting glucose in mmol/L × fasting insulin in microunits/mL ÷ 22.5). Insulin resistance is present if the index is ≥ 3.0 when measured more than 14 days post stroke. In one recent study non-diabetic TIA or stroke patients with insulin resistance had a lower subsequent incidence of diabetes or recurrent stroke/MI if treated with pioglitazone.[15] However, this was accompanied by a higher risk of edema and bone fracture, so such treatment should be individualized.

4. LIFESTYLE MODIFICATION

Lifestyle modification is an important part of the control of blood pressure, lipids, and glucose.

- Stop smoking. This is one of the most important things patients can do to prevent not only ischemic stroke but also heart disease, lung cancer, head and neck cancer, etc.
- Based on results of the PREDIMED trial,[16] the Mediterranean-style diet is recommended for secondary stroke prevention. Refer patients to a dietician who can educate them about this diet and the diabetic diet or a low-sodium diet if indicated.
- More exercise. Counsel the patient to adopt a less sedentary lifestyle and participate in even moderate exercise. Forty minutes, five times per week, is optimal.
- Estrogen in the form of hormonal contraceptives or hormone replacement therapy should be avoided in most cases.[17-19]

• Drugs of abuse and alcohol should be avoided and discouraged, especially vasoactive drugs such as cocaine and amphetamines. There are conflicting data on alcohol use. Data suggest that more than one drink per day (women) and more than two drinks per day (men) should be avoided. Moderate red wine consumption has been associated with lower vascular disease risk.

■ Antiplatelets and Anticoagulants

ANTIPLATELETS

Current acute ischemic stroke guidelines recommend aspirin started within 24–48 hours of stroke onset.[13] This is a generic "one size fits all" recommendation for all ischemic stroke patients. The guidelines do not specify a dose. Long-term aspirin therapy results in a ~20% relative risk reduction (RRR) of secondary stroke/other vascular events.[20]

There are alternatives to aspirin that include:

• **Clopidogrel (Plavix)** – May be slightly better than aspirin in preventing vascular events, particularly in patients with peripheral vascular disease, and better tolerated. However, the drug must be converted in the stomach to its active metabolite by cytochrome P450 2C19 (CYP2C19), and patients with an allele of the *CYP2C19* gene that results in loss of function may be resistant. CYP2C19 activity can be assessed by a blood test, but using this test to guide therapy, while logical, has not yet been proven to improve outcomes.

• **Aspirin/dipyridamole ER (Aggrenox, Asasantin)** – Two trials showed this combination to be 30% better than aspirin alone.[21,22] In another, aspirin/dipyridamole was comparable to clopidogrel but caused a slightly higher risk of bleeding.[23] Headache is a frequent side effect.

• **Prasugrel** (similar to clopidogrel but without dependence on CYP2C19 activity) or **ticagrelor** may be useful (but more expensive) alternatives, but to date they have not been sufficiently studied in stroke patients to be certain of long-term safety and superiority over aspirin or clopidogrel. Ticagrelor is an antiplatelet agent that reversibly interacts with the platelet P2Y12 ADP-receptor to prevent signal transduction and platelet activation. In the SOCRATES trial, patients with high-risk TIA or ischemic stroke with low NIHSS (< 6) were randomized to aspirin (300 mg load followed by 100 mg) versus ticagrelor (180 mg load, 90 mg BID for 90 days).[24] In prespecified subgroup analyses, there was benefit of ticagrelor in patients with stroke of atherosclerotic etiology and in aspirin-naïve patients.[24,25]

- **Cilostazol** is used mainly for intermittent claudication in patients with peripheral artery disease. Controlled trials in Asian patients have found that cilostazol is effective for preventing cerebral infarction compared to placebo, but no better than aspirin.[26] Bleeding was slightly less with cilostazol but headache, diarrhea, dizziness, and tachycardia were more frequent. As yet there are no high-quality data regarding the use of cilostazol for secondary stroke prevention in non-Asian ethnic groups.

- **Triflusal** is an antiplatelet agent that is structurally related to aspirin. It is available in some European and Latin American countries, but is considered investigational in the United States. A meta-analysis of four trials showed that the effectiveness of triflusal was similar to aspirin at preventing vascular events after stroke, and it had a lower rate of hemorrhagic complications.[27]

Dual Antiplatelet Therapy

Recurrent stroke events are more prevalent in the first few weeks after TIA or stroke. Recent data suggest that, in certain patient populations, dual antiplatelet therapy (DAPT) may be superior to single-agent treatment for prevention of such early stroke recurrence. Therefore, there is a growing trend to recommend DAPT for the first several weeks in many acute ischemic stroke patients.

- In patients with severe intracranial stenosis, SAMMPRIS showed that "aggressive" medical therapy which included aspirin 325 mg +

clopidogrel 75 mg for 90 days was superior to intracranial stenting, and also superior to historical controls that received either single antiplatelet therapy or anticoagulation.[28]

- In patients with non-cardioembolic TIA and mild strokes, recent large studies have supported the benefit of DAPT. CHANCE showed better results with clopidogrel (300 mg load followed by 75 mg daily) + aspirin 75 mg compared to aspirin alone, when started within 24 hours and continued for 21 days in Asian patients.[29] POINT showed better results with clopidogrel (600 mg load followed by 75 mg daily) + aspirin up to 325 mg compared to aspirin alone when started within 12 hours and continued for 90 days in European and American patients.[30]

- Prolonged treatment with DAPT results in higher rates of bleeding without benefit of greater stroke prevention.[30–33]

Based on these data, in our practice, we start with aspirin 81 or 325 mg in most non-cardioembolic ischemic stroke patients. In patients with TIA and mild strokes, we initiate DAPT with aspirin 81 mg plus clopidogrel (300 mg load followed by 75 mg) for 21 days. In line with the SAMMPRIS protocol, we continue aspirin 325 mg and clopidogrel 75 mg for 3 months in patients with severe intracranial atherosclerosis. In other perceived "higher-risk" subgroups – those with significant extracranial atherosclerosis or recurrent strokes despite single AP therapy – we may use DAPT for 21–90 days. We might recommend continued DAPT in patients with severe atherosclerotic narrowing or post stenting. We will not use DAPT in patients with hemorrhagic transformation of their infarct, multiple microbleeds, or other perceived increased risk of bleeding.

The entire area of "personalization" of antiplatelet therapy is one of active investigation, and these recommendations will undoubtedly change over the next several years. However, at present, we do not use platelet assays or genotyping to guide initial antiplatelet therapy.

ANTICOAGULANTS

Acute anticoagulation with heparin or an alternative has been addressed in Chapter 3. Here we consider choices for long-term secondary stroke prevention that you should consider after the work-up has been complete. The conditions are listed below more or less in order of the frequency you will encounter them. Anticoagulants most often used include warfarin (Coumadin) or one of the newer direct oral anticoagulants (DOACs), namely the direct thrombin inhibitor dabigatran, or one of the factor Xa inhibitors rivaroxaban, apixaban, or edoxaban. The decision to go with warfarin or a DOAC should be individualized, but the trend is to use DOACs, for several reasons:

- Multiple trials show that DOACs are as effective as and probably safer than warfarin.[34] There have been no "head-to-head" studies comparing the various DOACs. Rivaroxaban is the only one that can be dosed once daily; reading "between the lines" in the various studies, data suggest that apixaban may provide the best safety profile, and that dabigatran may provide the best efficacy profile.

- All DOACs provide effective anticoagulation within hours, thereby shortening hospital stay and obviating the need for "bridging."

- DOACs are easy to dose, with only slight adjustment for age or renal insufficiency.

- Cost is less of an issue than when DOACs were first marketed, and they are probably no more costly over the long term when considering their better safety/efficacy profile and absence of INR monitoring.

- There are now reversal agents available for both direct thrombin inhibitors and Xa inhibitors.

- The main disadvantage of DOACs is that there is no way to determine the level of anticoagulation by an accurate and quick point-of-care test. Therefore, for patients with severe clotting tendency where you want to be absolutely sure the patient remains anticoagulated, warfarin may be a better choice as long as the patient is willing and able to have frequent INR monitoring.

For most of the following, the use of warfarin or a DOAC can be considered based on either randomized trials (level A) or consensus recommendations (level C). However, except for those with class I evidence (i.e., where there is general agreement with anticoagulant use), either antiplatelet drugs or an anticoagulant can be used.

- Atrial fibrillation, except for "lone AF" (see below) (class I evidence).
- Critical extracranial carotid stenosis, string sign or total occlusion, especially if intraluminal thrombus is seen.
- Basilar thrombosis/stenosis.
- Arterial dissection.
- Other "embologenic" cardiac conditions:
  - rheumatic valvular disease or mechanical valve (class I evidence)
  - low left ventricular ejection fraction (< 30%)
  - akinesis or severe hypokinesis of left-ventricle segments (especially anterior wall or apex)
  - stroke soon after myocardial infarction, especially if mural thrombus is identified on TTE
  - aortic atheroma > 4 mm
- Coagulopathy, especially if history of venous thrombosis or pulmonary embolism.
- Cerebral venous sinus thrombosis.

■ Atrial Fibrillation

Atrial fibrillation (AF) is a frequent cause of stroke, especially in the elderly. A great deal is known about the prevention of stroke due to AF, and effective treatment is available.

DETECTION

The chance of detecting AF is greatest in proximity to the stroke, so careful scrutiny of any prehospital or ED ECGs is useful. Up to one-third of patients with stroke due to AF are in normal sinus rhythm on admission and may require prolonged cardiac monitoring to establish the diagnosis. If embolic stroke is suspected, continuous telemetry during the acute hospitalization is indicated. Occult AF can be detected with long-term monitoring using either a surface or implanted cardiac loop recorder. The optimal duration of extended monitoring is debatable. Multiple studies have shown that occult AF will be found in roughly 10% additional patients with monitoring up to 6 months post stroke, with most of those events occurring during the first month.[35] Recent studies have shown that extended monitoring will yield AF in 12–16% of patients with cryptogenic strokes within the first 12 months.[36,37] The importance of finding a brief episode of AF 6 months after a stroke is uncertain.

In patients in whom an embolic source is suspected based on imaging or other clinical features, we usually recommend monitoring for at least 1 month, using at minimum surface recording. Among patients with higher suspicion for AF, including patients with left atrial enlargement and patients with recurrent embolic stroke of undetermined source, an implantable device is reasonable. In the future, "wearable" devices will be more widely employed, such as the recently marketing Apple watch.

An important area of ongoing research is whether there are other structural or functional atrial abnormalities, but without AF, that might be associated with embolic stroke.

IN THE ACUTE STROKE SETTING

Acute stroke recurrence rate estimates vary; the best data suggest roughly 4% stroke recurrence in 14 days.

Therefore, there is no reason to rush to anticoagulate after an AF-related stroke. Wait 48–96 hours after a major stroke and repeat the CT (or MRI) first to exclude hemorrhagic transformation.

Guidelines suggest starting anticoagulation within 2 weeks;[13] optimal timing is unknown and is being studied in RCTs. Generally our recommendation is to be guided by the CT or MRI appearance of the infarcted region and to delay until cerebral edema or hemorrhagic transformation stabilizes and begins to subside. Aspirin can be given in the interim.

NATURAL HISTORY OF CHRONIC ATRIAL FIBRILLATION

- Valvular atrial fibrillation: stroke risk ~17 × that of controls.
- Non-valvular atrial fibrillation: stroke risk 6 × controls or ~5% per year.

Risk Stratification

- Low risk – "lone" atrial fibrillation, age < 60, none of the risk factors listed below, and no history of TIA, stroke, or other embolic event: 0.5% stroke risk per year.
- Moderate and high risk – variable combinations of age > 75, female sex, decreased left ventricular function, hypertension, diabetes, vascular disease, and previous cardioembolism: up to 10% stroke risk per year (see table of CHA_2DS_2-VASc score in Appendix 7).
  - Prior stroke/TIA/embolism: > 10% stroke risk per year.
  - So, by definition, any atrial fibrillation patient with embolic stroke or TIA is considered "high risk."
  - Age > 80: > 7% per year.

- Echocardiographic risk features include left ventricular dysfunction, left atrial enlargement or clot, mitral annular calcification, spontaneous echo contrast.

TREATMENT OF CHRONIC ATRIAL FIBRILLATION

The choice of antiplatelet therapy versus warfarin or DOAC depends on the risk of stroke, but as pointed out previously, a patient who has had a TIA or stroke automatically has enough risk to justify chronic anticoagulation. See the discussion of anticoagulants in the previous section to help guide your choice of warfarin or DOAC. As in all situations, the benefit of treatment must be balanced against the risks. The problem is that the very patients who have the highest risk of recurrent stroke – frail, elderly patients – are also the ones with the highest risk of treatment complications.

Anticoagulation results in a reduction of stroke risk to ~2% per year, or ~60% relative risk reduction compared to aspirin.

Major bleeding risk is 1.5–3.5% per year. The risk of bleeding increases with recent hemorrhage, falling, advanced age, alcohol binge, closed head injury, liver disease, aspirin, NSAIDs, cancer, and uncontrolled hypertension. Also, underlying amyloid angiopathy or microbleeds on MRI also confer increased risk. However, currently there are insufficient data to establish an imaging threshold for excluding a patient from anticoagulation. The HAS-BLED score is useful for assessing bleeding risk (see Appendix 7).

Alternatives to anticoagulation include ablation or atrial occlusive devices. The Watchman device has been approved by the FDA, and studies show it is as effective as warfarin in preventing strokes.[38] We expect that these approaches will become more widely utilized in patients who have contraindications or do not tolerate long-term anticoagulation.

■ Carotid Stenosis

Carotid stenosis is also one of the better-studied causes of stroke for which specific therapy is available. There is a large body of literature on carotid endarterectomy (CEA) and carotid stenting (CAS).

SYMPTOMATIC INTERNAL CAROTID STENOSIS (70–99% BY NASCET CRITERIA OF ANGIOGRAPHIC STENOSIS)

CEA is beneficial compared to medical therapy.[39]

- In NASCET, 2-year risk of ipsilateral stroke was 8.6% in the surgical group and 24.5% in the medical group (RRR 65%, ARR 16%, NNT 6 to prevent 1 stroke in 2 years).
- It is most beneficial to those who have highest risk of subsequent stroke: those who had hemispheric symptoms (compared to ocular symptoms), tandem extracranial and intracranial disease, and those without apparent collaterals.
- Perioperative risk was 5.8% overall, and was higher for those with contralateral internal carotid occlusion and those with intraluminal thrombus, but those high-risk patients still received benefit.

SYMPTOMATIC STENOSIS (50–69%)

Benefit of CEA is marginal.

- 5-year risk of any ipsilateral stroke was 15.7% surgical versus 22.2% medical treatment (ARR 7%, $p = 0.045$).
- No benefit in preventing disabling strokes.

- Women and those whose symptoms were limited to transient monocular blindness did not benefit.
- 6.7% 1-month surgical morbidity and mortality in NASCET.

ASYMPTOMATIC STENOSIS

The benefit of treating asymptomatic carotid stenosis is much less clear compared to symptomatic disease, and is currently being re-evaluated.

Two large randomized trials carried out 15–25 years ago showed that CEA for stenosis ≥ 60~70% reduces ipsilateral ischemic stroke compared to medical therapy.[40,41]

- ACAS showed that the 5-year risk was 5.1% for surgical versus 11.0% for medical therapy.
- The results were confirmed by the ACST trial, which showed 5-year stroke risk of 6.4% for surgical versus 11.8% for medical therapy.
- The overall subsequent risk is smaller than that for symptomatic carotid stenosis. The absolute risk reduction (ARR) is about 1% per year, with NNT 17–19 to prevent 1 ipsilateral ischemic stroke in 5 years.
- The perioperative risk was 2.3% in ACAS and 3.1% in ACST.

One of the main reasons for re-evaluating CEA and CAS for asymptomatic stenosis is that the relatively small benefit seen in the studies carried out in the past might be erased by the improvement in medical therapy that has occurred in the interim. This "aggressive" medical therapy includes rigorous control of all the various risk factors discussed earlier in this chapter.

CREST-2 is two independent ongoing parallel trials in patients with asymptomatic carotid stenosis > 70%:

- Best medical management with and without CEA
- Best medical management with and without CAS

In the interim, while awaiting the results of CREST-2, the best asymptomatic patients for CEA or CAS would be those who are on aggressive medical management of their risk factors and have the highest stroke risk (stenosis > 70%) and the lowest risk of complications (younger age, fewer comorbidities, favorable anatomy), again keeping in mind that women do not benefit as much as men.

CAROTID STENTING VERSUS ENDARTERECTOMY

Both CAS and CEA are options for dealing with carotid stenosis.

- A number of small studies suggested that CAS was an effective alternative to CEA.
- CREST was published in 2010, comparing CEA to CAS in both symptomatic (> 50%) and asymptomatic (> 60%) stenosis.[42]
  - The two interventions were more or less equivalent for both symptomatic and asymptomatic disease.
  - The rate of subsequent vascular events over 10 years was very low in both groups.
  - There was a higher risk of perioperative MI in patients undergoing CEA, and a higher risk of perioperative stroke in those having CAS.
  - There was also an age interaction, with patients > 70 years old doing better with CEA.
- These results were more or less confirmed in the ACT-1 trial.[43]

In summary, CAS can be considered as an alternative to CEA in younger patients, and in symptomatic patients where the stenosis is hard to reach surgically, where there are medical comorbidities that increase the risk of surgery, or in cases of post-radiation or postoperative stenoses.

WHEN CAN YOU DO SURGERY OR STENTING AFTER A STROKE?

Reperfusing an area of recent stroke might lead to hyperperfusion or even hemorrhage. However, because the risk of recurrent stroke is highest in the first few weeks, combined data from the NASCET and ECST trials show that the benefit of CEA is greatest when it is performed within 2 weeks of symptoms.[44,45] In the era of endovascular thrombectomy (EVT), it is not unusual to stent an associated carotid stenosis at the time of EVT. Therefore, the timing of CEA or CAS should be individualized; it should be carried out as soon as possible once the patient's hemodynamic, neurological, and brain imaging status has stabilized.

■ Carotid Occlusion

Carotid occlusion can cause a stroke by two mechanisms:
• Hemodynamic reduction of flow
• Embolism into the downstream cerebral circulation
These two mechanisms can often be distinguished by the appearance of the stroke on MRI, and by perfusion studies. Hemodynamic strokes will have a "watershed" distribution of infarction and reduced flow in the distal beds of the MCA, ACA, and PCA, while emboli will have a classical embolic distribution of infarction and reduced flow in the branches of these vessels.

Carotid occlusion patients are at high risk for recurrent stroke by either mechanism.

Some patients with acute distal intracranial carotid occlusion can benefit from urgent thrombectomy (see Chapter 6). If the proximal ICA is occluded, this can be stented at the same time. However, in general, patients with symptomatic acute complete carotid occlusion are managed conservatively with careful maintenance of cerebral perfusion by cautious blood-pressure control, antiplatelet drugs, and risk-factor reduction.

A randomized trial in patients with chronic carotid occlusion evaluating extracranial–intracranial bypass surgery versus medical therapy was terminated because of no benefit.[46] Such bypass surgery is now largely restricted to patients with distal carotid occlusion due to moyamoya disease.

If bypass is considered, there are several measurement methods for risk stratification by hemodynamic reserve:

- Single-photon emission CT (SPECT) with acetazolamide (Diamox) challenge
- Positron-emission tomography (PET) with oxygen extraction fraction
- Transcranial Doppler (TCD) with breath-holding index (BHI):
  - normal BHI ≥ 0.69 → < 10% ipsilateral stroke in 2 years
  - impaired BHI < 0.69 → 40% ipsilateral stroke in 2 years

■ Intracranial Stenosis

Severe intracranial stenosis is associated with high rates of recurrent stroke.

The WASID trial compared warfarin (target INR 2–3) with aspirin (1300 mg daily) in patients with symptomatic intracranial stenosis of 50–99%.[47] The trial was stopped early owing to statistically significant higher death and major hemorrhage rates in the warfarin group. However, the authors did find that combined stroke rates in the territory of the stenotic artery at 1 and 2 years were 11% and 14% respectively in patients with < 70% stenosis, and the 1-year stroke rate was 7% versus 18% in those with > 70% stenosis. Due to high rates of stroke with medical therapy alone, researchers have been looking for other ways to reduce stroke rates, such as with angioplasty and stenting.

SAMMPRIS randomized patients similar to the highest-risk patients in WASID (those with > 70% intracranial stenosis) to "aggressive" medical therapy with or without stenting.[28] Medical therapy included coaching the patient about medication compliance to control risk factors, as well as DAPT for 3 months. Surprisingly, the study was stopped prematurely because medical therapy was superior to intracranial stenting, and also superior to historical matched WASID controls that received either single antiplatelet therapy or anticoagulation.

These results show the power of optimal atherosclerotic risk-factor management and DAPT for stroke prevention in patients at highest risk of stroke recurrence. They have galvanized a major shift in our stroke program to help ensure that patients adhere to optimal secondary stroke prevention strategies. Intracranial stenting is rarely carried out, in light of the SAMMPRIS results, unless the patient continues to have symptoms despite aggressive medical management.

■ Lacunar Strokes

Lacunar strokes, also known as small-vessel disease or small-vessel occlusion, account for approximately 20–30% of strokes. They are due to obstruction of penetrating end arteries off major intracranial arteries (MCA, basilar artery, PCA, ACA, and posterior communicating artery). These infarcts are < 15 mm in diameter.

ARE ALL SMALL SUBCORTICAL STROKES < 15 mm LACUNAR STROKES (i.e., DUE TO SMALL-VESSEL DISEASE)?

No, they are not: 12% of small basal ganglia and 34% of centrum semiovale infarcts have a cardioembolic source, and 19% of small basal ganglia and 53% of centrum semiovale infarcts have large-artery occlusive disease.[48] Some are larger than 15 mm and are clearly not in a distribution of a single small arteriole. Not all lacunar syndromes (see below) are caused by small strokes. Therefore, even a "lacunar-looking" stroke, especially if it does not fit into a classic syndrome or appearance, warrants careful work-up for large-artery atherosclerosis and an embolic source.

WHAT CAUSES LACUNAR STROKES?

Lipohyalinosis is the classic pathology, but atherosclerosis is also a common cause for small-vessel branch occlusion. Seen from an epidemiological standpoint, hypertension is the only consistent risk factor, whereas the contributions of diabetes mellitus, smoking, or hyperlipidemia are smaller.

LACUNAR SYNDROMES AND THEIR LOCALIZATION (SEE ALSO APPENDIX 4)

- **Pure motor hemiparesis**– corona radiata, anterior or posterior limb of internal capsule, pons, and medullary pyramid
- **Pure sensory stroke** – ventral posterior thalamus
- **Sensorimotor stroke** – thalamus, corona radiata
- **Ataxic hemiparesis** – not well localizing: pons, corona radiata, anterior or posterior limb of internal capsule, lentiform nucleus, cerebellum
- **Dysarthria/clumsy hand** – anterior limb of internal capsule, genu, pons

FLUCTUATIONS

Lacunar syndromes often fluctuate and mislead the clinician into anticipating a good outcome only to find the patient with a severe deficit the next day. "Lacunar TIAs" may occur in up to 20% of patients immediately preceding the completed infarct. We

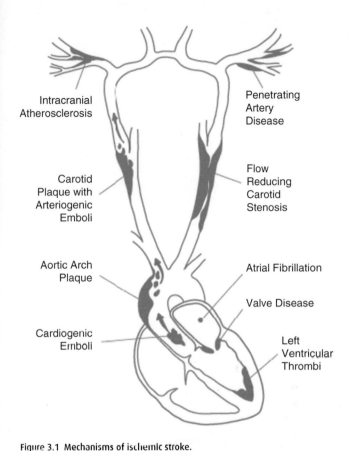

Figure 3.1 Mechanisms of ischemic stroke.
Source: Albers GW, Amarenco P, Easton JD, Sacco RL, Teal P. Antithrombotic and thrombolytic therapy for ischemic stroke: the Seventh ACCP Conference on Antithrombotic and Thrombolytic Therapy. *Chest* 2004; 126 (3 suppl): 483S–512S.[6] Reproduced with permission.

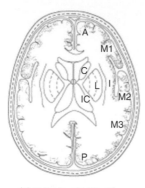 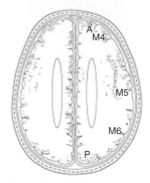

(a) at the level of basal
ganglia and thalamus

(a) at the level just rostral to
basal ganglia

Figure 4.1 ASPECTS template.
Source: Barber PA, Demchuk AM, Zhang J, Buchan AM. Validity and reliability of a quantitative computed tomography score in predicting outcome of hyperacute stroke before thrombolytic therapy. ASPECTS Study Group. Alberta Stroke Programme Early CT Score. *Lancet* 2000; 355: 1670–1674.[5] Reproduced with permission from Elsevier.

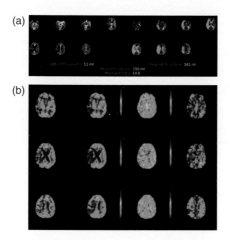

Figure 4.3 RAPID map. For further information, see: Albers GW. Use of imaging to select patients for late window endovascular therapy. *Stroke* 2018; 49: 2256–2260.[14]

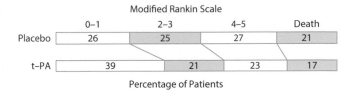

Figure 5.2 Three-month outcome in NINDS tPA study by modified Rankin scale (mRS).
Source: National Institute of Neurological Disorders and Stroke rt-PA Stroke Study Group.
Tissue plasminogen activator for acute ischemic stroke. *N Engl J Med* 1995; 333: 1581–1587.[1]
Reproduced with permission.

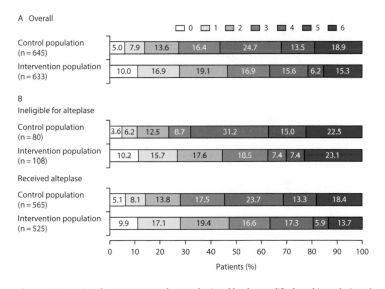

**Figure 6.1 Functional outcome at 90 days as depicted by the modified Rankin scale (mRS)
score distribution in endovascular therapy compared with medical management.**
Source: Goyal M, Menon BK, van Zwam WH, *et al.*; HERMES collaborators. Endovascular
thrombectomy after large-vessel ischaemic stroke: a meta-analysis of individual patient data
from five randomised trials. *Lancet* 2016; 387: 1723–1731.[22] Reproduced with permission.

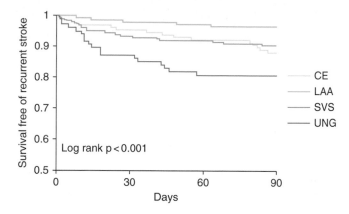

Figure 7.1 Stroke recurrence risk by stroke mechanism.
Source: Lovett JK, Coull AJ, Rothwell PM. Early risk of recurrence by subtype of ischemic stroke in population-based incidence studies. *Neurology* 2004; 62: 569–573.[12] Reproduced with permission.

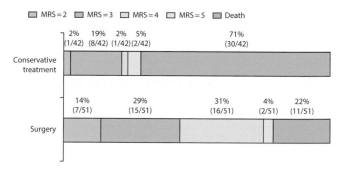

Figure 7.2 Pooled analysis comparing outcomes of decompressive hemicraniectomy and control groups among patients with malignant MCA stroke under the age of 60.
Source: Vahedi K, Hofmeijer J, Juettler E, *et al.* Early decompressive surgery in malignant infarction of the middle cerebral artery: a pooled analysis of three randomised controlled trials. *Lancet Neurol* 2007; 6: 215–222.[16] Reproduced with permission.

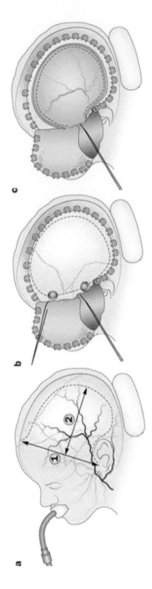

Figure 7.4 Technique for decompressive hemicraniectomy and duratomy.
Source: Kolias AG, Kirkpatrick PJ, Hutchinson PJ. Decompressive craniectomy: past, present and future. *Nat Rev Neurol* 2013; 9: 405–415.[18] Reproduced with permission.

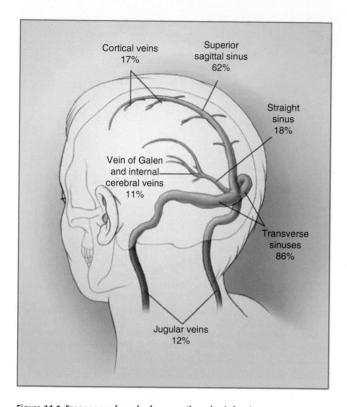

Figure 11.1 Frequency of cerebral venous thrombosis by site.
Adapted from: Stam J. Thrombosis of the cerebral veins and sinuses. *N Engl J Med* 2005; 352: 1791–1798.[2]

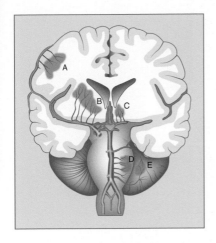

Figure 12.1 Location of hemorrhages: (A) penetrating cortical branches of the anterior, middle, or posterior cerebral arteries; (B) basal ganglia, originating from ascending lenticulostriate branches of the middle cerebral artery; (C) the thalamus, originating from ascending thalamogeniculate branches of the posterior cerebral artery; (D) the pons, originating from paramedian branches of the basilar artery; and (E) the cerebellum, originating from penetrating branches of the posterior inferior, anterior inferior, or superior cerebellar arteries.

Source: Qureshi AI, Tuhrim S, Broderick JP, *et al.* Spontaneous intracerebral hemorrhage. *N Engl J Med* 2001; 344: 1450–1460.[2] Copyright © 2001 Massachusetts Medical Society. Reproduced with permission from the Massachusetts Medical Society.

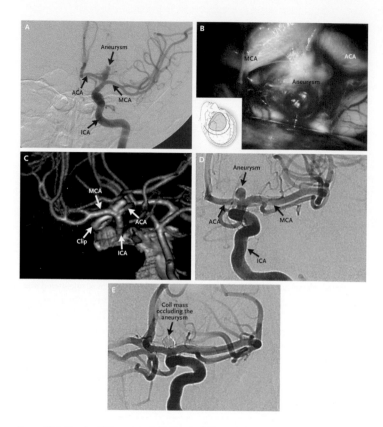

Figure 13.1 Terminal ICA aneurysm before and after treatment. Panels A, B, C are from a patient who underwent clipping (respectively: DSA pre-treatment; at the time of clipping; post-clipping CTA with reconstruction). Panels D and E refer to another patient who underwent coiling (respectively: before and after treatment).

Source: Lawton MT, Vates GE. Subarachnoid hemorrhage. *N Engl J Med* 2017; 377: 257–266.[6]

prospectively examined a series of 90 subcortical stroke patients.[49] Deterioration occurred in about 40%, mainly in the first 24 hours; only about one-third of those who deteriorated then recovered to their pre-deterioration status. Deterioration was not explained by fluctuations in blood pressure, glucose, or treatment (or non-treatment) with antiplatelet or antithrombotic agents, though these fluctuations were slightly more frequent in patients treated with tPA. In our experience, no particular intervention seems to reverse deterioration. Appropriate treatment probably awaits a better understanding of how to arrest or reverse the underlying lipohyalinosis of the penetrating vessel.

TREATMENT

Treatment is control of risk factors, in particular careful control of blood pressure avoiding fluctuations. Long-term careful antihypertensive treatment reduces the burden of lacunar strokes. Single antiplatelet therapy is usually sufficient unless there are multiple acute infarcts or significant underlying large-artery atherosclerosis. The SPS3 study showed that long-term DAPT resulted in no benefit and more bleeding in these patients.[31]

■ Cervical Arterial Dissection

Arterial dissection is probably an under-recognized stroke mechanism.

PATHOLOGY

Dissection occurs because of an intimal tear in the vessel wall and the formation of an intramural hematoma, sometimes associated with a pseudoaneurysm. Flow may be obstructed by compression of the lumen by the wall hematoma, or by intraluminal clot. Distal embolization from the area of injury downstream into the intracranial circulation is probably the most common stroke mechanism.

In the internal carotid artery, dissection usually occurs about 2 cm distal to the carotid bifurcation, and in the vertebral artery at the C1–2 level where the artery leaves the transverse canal of the axis bone. Intracranial dissections can also occur but are less common.

Dissections of the intracranial vertebral arteries are especially prone to subarachnoid hemorrhage.

Neck or head trauma and chiropractic manipulation are precipitating factors. Motor vehicle accidents with whiplash or seatbelt injuries to the neck are probably the most common cause seen in most hospitals. However, many people with cervical artery dissections do not have clear precipitating events.

Fibromuscular dysplasia and heritable arteriopathies such as Ehlers–Danlos syndrome predispose to arterial dissections, but most individuals do not have underlying arterial pathology.

DIAGNOSIS

The usual presenting symptoms do not differ much from typical TIA or stroke, except that prominent neck, facial, or head pain in a patient without strong risk factors for vascular disease points toward the diagnosis. Horner syndrome may occur because of injury to sympathetic fibers lying on the outside of the carotid artery wall. Subarachnoid hemorrhage can occur if the dissection occurs or extends intracranially, because there are only two layers in the vessel wall, compared to three extracranially.

TESTING

When dissection is suspected, diagnostic testing should go beyond routine carotid ultrasound and MR angiography. Carotid ultrasound may miss a dissection since they are usually rostral to the bifurcation. MRA may miss a subtle intimal tear and flap.

Better diagnostic tests:

- **MRI T1 sequence with fat suppression of the neck** – Talk to your radiologist to be sure he or she knows that dissection is suspected. Hematoma in false lumen is bright.
- **CT angiogram** – A good CTA can give information similar to DSA.
- **Digital subtraction angiogram (DSA)** – Finds a characteristic tapering lumen, rarely pseudoaneurysm, in locations usually not associated with atherosclerosis. Though considered a gold standard, sometimes it is not clear whether the abnormality is due to dissection or atherosclerosis.
- **CT or MRI brain** should be scrutinized for subarachnoid blood if intracranial extension of the dissection is possible.

Several diagnostic methodologies might be necessary before you can conclude that the underlying problem is a dissection.

THERAPY

Anticoagulation has been the traditional medical therapy, since the mechanism of cerebral infarction is probably most often thromboembolism, though there are no randomized trials to support anticoagulation. In the CADISS trial, patients with cervical dissection were randomized to antiplatelet therapy or anticoagulation.[50] There was no benefit of anticoagulation over antiplatelet therapy in this trial. The risk of stroke/TIA recurrence is low (~1.5% per year), and it occurs most often in the first few days.[51] Therefore, antiplatelet therapy without anticoagulation seems just as reasonable, especially if the diagnosis is not established right away. We generally recommend anticoagulation for the first few days after dissection, especially if an intraluminal thrombus is visualized, and then transition to antiplatelet therapy. Anticoagulation should be withheld if there is any subarachnoid hemorrhage. Most of the time, dissected arteries heal over time, sometimes leaving variable degrees of residual stenosis or a pseudoaneurysm.

Sometimes dissection requires endovascular treatment, though intervention is not needed in most cases. The indications for intervention include expanding pseudoaneurysm, recurrent symptoms due to hemodynamically significant stenosis, or intracranial vertebral artery dissection with subarachnoid hemorrhage.

■ Patent Foramen Ovale

Patent foramen ovale (PFO) is very prevalent, and the role of PFO in pathophysiology and prevention of stroke has been controversial. However, recent large prospective studies have clarified appropriate management.

RELATION TO STROKE

- PFO is detected in 20–30% of the general population.
- PFO is more prevalent (30–50%) among stroke patients who are young and do not have other causes of stroke (cryptogenic, age < 50).
- Recurrent stroke in patients with PFO and no other obvious cause who are treated with antiplatelet agents is very low, similar to asymptomatic carotid stenosis (~1% per year).

PFO is more likely causally related to the stroke when the PFO is large (e.g., a larger right-to-left shunt) and associated with an atrial septal aneurysm.[52] PFO is less likely a causal factor for stroke when it is found in a person who has known atherosclerosis or another known stroke mechanism, or is elderly (> 60).

The proposed mechanism relating PFO to ischemic stroke is "paradoxical embolism." Venous thrombus in systemic venous circulation bypasses the pulmonary circulation and embolizes to the brain. Finding deep venous thrombosis in the lower extremities (by ultrasound) or in the pelvic veins (by MRI), or detecting hypercoagulability (factor V Leiden, prothrombin gene mutation, anticardiolipin antibodies, etc.), would support this mechanism.

TREATMENT

Initial studies of PFO closure were inconclusive, but three recent studies with more careful patient selection, more statistical power, and prolonged follow-up have clarified management and have shown significant reduction in recurrent stroke with a low incidence of complications, mainly new atrial fibrillation.[53-55] Therefore, we recommend PFO closure in patients < 60 years old with a sizable right-to-left shunt who have a non-lacunar stroke without proximal arterial stenosis or cardioembolic source.

References

1. Chobanian AV, Bakris GL, Black HR, *et al.* The Seventh Report of the Joint National Committee on Prevention, Detection, Evaluation, and Treatment of High Blood Pressure: the JNC 7 report. *JAMA* 2003; 289: 2560–2572.
2. SHEP Cooperative Research Group. Prevention of stroke by antihypertensive drug treatment in older persons with isolated systolic hypertension. Final results of the Systolic Hypertension in the Elderly Program (SHEP). *JAMA* 1991; 265: 3255–3264.
3. Yusuf S, Sleight P, Pogue J, *et al.*; Heart Outcomes Prevention Evaluation Study Investigators. Effects of an angiotensin-converting-enzyme inhibitor, ramipril, on cardiovascular events in high-risk patients. *N Engl J Med* 2000; 342: 145–153.

4. PROGRESS Collaborative Group. Randomised trial of a perindopril-based blood-pressure-lowering regimen among 6,105 individuals with previous stroke or transient ischaemic attack. *Lancet* 2001; 358: 1033–1041.

5. ALLHAT Collaborative Research Group. Major outcomes in high-risk hypertensive patients randomized to angiotensin-converting enzyme inhibitor or calcium channel blocker vs diuretic. The Antihypertensive and Lipid-Lowering Treatment to Prevent Heart Attack Trial (ALLHAT). *JAMA* 2002; 288: 2981–2997.

6. Dahlof B, Devereux RB, Kjeldsen SE, *et al.* Cardiovascular morbidity and mortality in the Losartan Intervention For Endpoint reduction in hypertension study (LIFE): a randomised trial against atenolol. *Lancet* 2002; 359: 995–1003.

7. Psaty BM, Lumley T, Furberg CD, *et al.* Health outcomes associated with various antihypertensive therapies used as first-line agents: a network meta-analysis. *JAMA* 2003; 289: 2534–2544.

8. Whelton PK, Carey RM, Aronow WS, *et al.* 2017 ACC/AHA/AAPA/ABC/ACPM/AGS/APhA/ASH/ASPC/NMA/PCNA guideline for the prevention, detection, evaluation, and management of high blood pressure in adults: executive summary: a report of the American College of Cardiology/American Heart Association Task Force on Clinical Practice Guidelines. *Circulation* 2018; 138: e426–e483. doi:10.1161/CIR.0000000000000597.

9. Wright JT, Williamson JD, Whelton PK, *et al.* A randomized trial of intensive versus standard blood-pressure control. *N Engl J Med* 2015; 373: 2103–2116.

10. Grundy SM, Stone NJ, Bailey AL, *et al.* AHA/ACC/AACVPR/AAPA/ABC/ACPM/ADA/AGS/APhA/ASPC/NLA/PCNA guideline on the management of blood cholesterol. A report of the American College of Cardiology/American Heart Association Task Force on Clinical Practice Guidelines. *Circulation* 2019; 139: e1046–e1081. doi:10.1161/CIR.0000000000000625.

11. Amarenco P, Bogousslavsky J, Callahan A, *et al.*; Stroke Prevention by Aggressive Reduction in Cholesterol Levels (SPARCL) Investigators.High-dose atorvastatin after stroke or transient ischemic attack. *N Engl J Med* 2006; 355: 549–559.

12. Heart Protection Study Collaborative Group. MRC/BHF Heart Protection Study of cholesterol lowering with simvastatin in 20 536 high-risk individuals: a randomised placebo-controlled trial. *Lancet* 2002; 360: 7–22.

13. Powers WJ, Rabinstein AA, Ackerson T, *et al.*; American Heart Association Stroke Council. 2018 guidelines for the early management of patients with acute ischemic stroke: a guideline for healthcare professionals from the American Heart Association/American Stroke Association. *Stroke* 2018; 49: e46–e110. doi:10.1161/STR.0000000000000158.

14. Bruno A, Durkalski VL, Hall CE, *et al.* The Stroke Hyperglycemia Insulin Network Effort (SHINE) trial protocol: a randomized, blinded, efficacy trial of standard vs. intensive hyperglycemia management in acute stroke. *Int J Stroke* 2014; 9: 246–251. doi:10.1111/ijs.12045.

15. Kernan WN, Viscoli CM, Furie KL, *et al.* Pioglitazone after ischemic stroke or transient ischemic attack. *N Engl J Med* 2016; 374: 1321–1331. doi:10.1056/NEJMoa1506930.

16. Estruch R, Ros E, Salas-Salvadó J, *et al.*; PREDIMED Study Investigators. Primary prevention of cardiovascular disease with a Mediterranean diet. *N Engl J Med* 2013; 368: 1279–1290. Corrected and republished in: *N Engl J Med* 2018; 378: e34.

17. Viscoli CM, Brass LM, Kernan WN, *et al.* A clinical trial of estrogen replacement therapy after ischemic stroke. *N Engl J Med* 2001; 345: 1243–1249.

18. Anderson GL, Limacher M, Assaf AR, *et al.* Effects of conjugated equine estrogen in postmenopausal women with hysterectomy: the Women's Health Initiative randomized controlled trial. *JAMA* 2004; 291: 1701–1712.

19. Rossouw JE, Anderson GL, Prentice RL, *et al.* Risks and benefits of estrogen plus progestin in healthy postmenopausal women: principal results from the Women's Health Initiative randomized controlled trial. *JAMA* 2002; 288: 321–333.

20. Antiplatelet Trialists' Collaboration. Collaborative overview of randomised trials of antiplatelet therapy. I: Prevention of death, myocardial infarction, and stroke by prolonged antiplatelet therapy in various categories of patients. *BMJ* 1994; 308: 81–106.

21. Diener HC, Cunha L, Forbes C, *et al.* European Stroke Prevention Study. 2. Dipyridamole and acetylsalicylic acid in the secondary prevention of stroke. *J Neurol Sci* 1996; 143: 1–13.

22. ESPS Group. The European Stroke Prevention Study (ESPS): principal end-points. *Lancet* 1987; 2: 1351–1354.

23. Sacco RL, Diener HC, Yusuf S, *et al.*; PRoFESS Study Group. Aspirin and extended-release dipyridamole versus clopidogrel for recurrent stroke. *N Engl J Med* 2008; 359: 1238–1251.

24. Johnston SC, Amarenco P, Albers GW, *et al.* Ticagrelor versus aspirin in acute stroke or transient ischemic attack. *N Engl J Med* 2016; 375: 35–43. doi:10.1056/NEJMoa1603060.

25. Amarenco P, Albers GW, Denison H, *et al.* Efficacy and safety of ticagrelor versus aspirin in acute stroke or transient ischaemic attack of atherosclerotic origin: a subgroup analysis of SOCRATES, a randomised, double-blind, controlled trial. *Lancet Neurol* 2017; 16: 301–310. doi:10.1016/S1474-4422(17)30038-8.

26. Dinicolantonio JJ, Lavie CJ, Fares H, *et al.* Meta-analysis of cilostazol versus aspirin for the secondary prevention of stroke. *Am J Cardiol* 2013; 112: 1230–1234. doi:10.1016/j.amjcard.2013.05.067.

27. Costa J, Ferro JM, Matias-Guiu J, Álvarez-Sabín J, Torres F. Triflusal for preventing serious vascular events in people at high risk. *Cochrane Database Syst Rev* 2005; (3): CD004296.

28. Chimowitz MI, Lynn MJ, Derdeyn CP, *et al.*; SAMMPRIS Trial Investigators. Stenting versus aggressive medical therapy for intracranial arterial stenosis. *N Engl J Med* 2011; 365: 993–1003.

29. Wang Y, Wang Y, Zhao X, *et al.*; CHANCE Investigators. Clopidogrel with aspirin in acute minor stroke or transient ischemic attack. *N Engl J Med* 2013; 369: 11–19. doi:10.1056/NEJMoa1215340.

30. Johnston SC, Easton JD, Farrant M, *et al.* Clopidogrel and aspirin in acute ischemic stroke and high-risk TIA. *N Engl J Med* 2018; 379: 215–225. doi:10.1056/NEJMoa1800410.

31. Benavente OR, Hart RG, McClure LA, *et al.*; SPS3 Investigators. Effects of clopidogrel added to aspirin in patients with recent lacunar stroke. *N Engl J Med* 2012; 367: 817–825. doi:10.1056/NEJMoa1204133.

32. Diener HC, Bogousslavsky J, Brass LM, *et al.* Aspirin and clopidogrel compared with clopidogrel alone after recent ischaemic stroke or transient ischaemic attack in high-risk patients (MATCH): randomised, double-blind, placebo-controlled trial. *Lancet* 2004; 364: 331–337.

33. Bhatt DL, Fox KA, Hacke W, *et al.* Clopidogrel and aspirin versus aspirin alone for the prevention of atherothrombotic events. *N Engl J Med* 2006; 354: 1706–1717.

34. van Es N, Coppens M, Schulman S, *et al.* Direct oral anticoagulants compared with vitamin K antagonists for acute venous thromboembolism: evidence from phase 3 trials. *Blood* 2014; 124: 1968–1975. doi:10.1182/blood-2014-04-571232.

35. Choe WC, Passman RS, Brachmann J, *et al.* A comparison of atrial fibrillation monitoring strategies after cryptogenic stroke (from the Cryptogenic Stroke and Underlying AF Trial). *Am J Cardiol* 2015; 116: 889–893. doi:10.1016/j.amjcard.2015.06.012.

36. Sanna T, Diener HC, Passman RS, *et al.* Cryptogenic stroke and underlying atrial fibrillation. *N Engl J Med* 2014; 370: 2478–2486.

37. Gladstone DJ, Spring M, Dorian P, *et al.* Atrial fibrillation in patients with cryptogenic stroke. *N Engl J Med* 2014; 370: 2467–2477.

38. Reddy VY, Doshi SK, Kar S, *et al.* 5-year outcomes after left atrial appendage closure: from the PREVAIL and PROTECT AF trials. *J Am Coll Cardiol* 2017; 70: 2964–2975. doi:10.1016/j.jacc.2017.10.021.

39. Barnett HJ, Taylor DW, Eliasziw M, *et al.*; North American Symptomatic Carotid Endarterectomy Trial Collaborators. Benefit of carotid endarterectomy in patients with symptomatic moderate or severe stenosis. *N Engl J Med* 1998; 339: 1415–1425.

40. Executive Committee for the Asymptomatic Carotid Atherosclerosis Study. Endarterectomy for asymptomatic carotid artery stenosis. *JAMA* 1995; 273: 1421–1428.

41. Halliday A, Mansfield A, Marro J, *et al.*; MRC Asymptomatic Carotid Surgery Trial (ACST) Collaborative Group. Prevention of disabling and fatal strokes by successful carotid endarterectomy in patients without recent neurological symptoms: randomised controlled trial. *Lancet* 2004; 363: 1491–1502.

42. Brott TG, Hobson RW, Howard G, *et al.*; CREST Investigators. Stenting versus endarterectomy for treatment of carotid-artery stenosis. *N Engl J Med* 2010; 363: 11–23.

43. Rosenfield K, Matsumura JS, Chaturvedi S, *et al.* Randomized trial of stent versus surgery for asymptomatic carotid stenosis. *N Engl J Med* 2016; 374: 1011–1020. doi:10.1056/NEJMoa1515706.

44. Rothwell PM, Eliasziw M, Gutnikov SA, *et al.* Endarterectomy for symptomatic carotid stenosis in relation to clinical subgroups and timing of surgery. *Lancet* 2004; 363: 915–924.

45. Rothwell PM, Eliasziw M, Gutnikov SA, *et al.* Sex difference in the effect of time from symptoms to surgery on benefit from carotid endarterectomy for transient ischemic attack and nondisabling stroke. *Stroke* 2004; 35: 2855–2861.

46. Grubb RL, Powers WJ, Derdeyn CP, *et al.* The carotid occlusion surgery study. *Neurosurg Focus* 2003; 14 (3): e9.

47. Chimowitz MI, Lynn MJ, Howlett-Smith H, *et al.*; Warfarin-Aspirin Symptomatic Intracranial Disease Trial Investigators. Comparison of warfarin and aspirin for symptomatic intracranial arterial stenosis. *N Engl J Med* 2005; 352: 1305–1316.

48. Yonemura K, Kimura K, Minematsu K, *et al.* Small centrum ovale infarcts on diffusion-weighted magnetic resonance imaging. *Stroke* 2002; 33: 1541–1544.

49. Vahidy FS, Hicks WJ, Acosta I, *et al.* Neurofluctuation in patients with subcortical ischemic stroke. *Neurology* 2014; 83: 398–405. doi:10.1212/WNL.0000000000000643.

50. Markus HS, Hayter E, Levi C, *et al.* Antiplatelet treatment compared with anticoagulation treatment for cervical artery dissection (CADISS): a randomised trial. CADISS trial investigators. *Lancet Neurol* 2015; 14: 361–367. doi:10.1016/S1474-4422(15)70018-9. Erratum in: *Lancet Neurol* 2015; 14: 566.

51. Touze E, Gauvrit JY, Moulin T, *et al.* Risk of stroke and recurrent dissection after a cervical artery dissection: a multicenter study. *Neurology* 2003; 61: 1347–1351.

52. Overell JR, Bone I, Lees KR. Interatrial septal abnormalities and stroke: a meta-analysis of case-control studies. *Neurology* 2000; 55: 1172–1179.

53. Mas JL, Derumeaux G, Guillon B, *et al.*; CLOSE Investigators. Patent foramen ovale closure or anticoagulation vs. antiplatelets after stroke. *N Engl J Med* 2017; 377: 1011–1021. doi:10.1056/NEJMoa1705915.

54. Saver JL, Carroll JD, Thaler DE, *et al.*; RESPECT Investigators. Long-term outcomes of patent foramen ovale closure or medical therapy after stroke. *N Engl J Med* 2017; 377: 1022–1032. doi:10.1056/NEJMoa1610057.

55. Søndergaard L, Kasner SE, Rhodes JF, *et al.*; Gore REDUCE Clinical Study Investigators. Patent foramen ovale closure or antiplatelet therapy for cryptogenic stroke. *N Engl J Med* 2017; 377: 1033–1042. doi:10.1056/NEJMoa1707404.

9

Transient Ischemic Attack

Transient neurological symptoms often present a difficult diagnostic dilemma. It is often difficult to tell if the transient symptoms were due to ischemia or due to something else (see Chapter 1). Usually, by the time the physician sees the patient, the neurological exam has returned to normal. On the other hand, it is critically important not to miss the diagnosis of transient ischemic attack (TIA). TIAs may provide an opportunity for physicians to intervene and prevent an ischemic stroke and subsequent disability, and must be taken seriously. The search for an etiology must be done expeditiously. Just as angina may serve as a warning for future myocardial infarction, a TIA is often a warning sign of an impending stroke.

■ Definition

A transient ischemic attack (TIA) is a brief episode of neurological dysfunction caused by focal brain or retinal ischemia, with clinical symptoms typically lasting less than 1 hour, and without evidence of acute infarction on brain imaging.[1]

■ Etiology

The causes are the same as for ischemic stroke. Determining the etiology of the TIA expeditiously and providing the appropriate treatment is very important, as it may prevent a future stroke. Examples include atrial fibrillation and symptomatic carotid stenosis.

■ Presentation

TIAs present the same way as an acute ischemic stroke. The only difference is that the symptoms and signs rapidly and completely resolve, usually within minutes. There is not a typical presentation – it depends on the vascular territory affected.

■ Differential Diagnosis

- Syncope – look for pre-syncopal symptoms.
- Seizure – ask about prior history of seizure, or if any of the following occurred with the event: shaking, clouding of consciousness, tongue-biting, incontinence.
- Migraine – be careful about attributing a TIA or stroke to migraine unless there is a clear history of previous migraine with focal features similar to this event.
- Vestibular dysfunction, vertigo.
- Anxiety, panic attack.
- Hypoglycemia.
- Drug intoxication.
- Mass such as tumor or subdural hematoma.
- Metabolic encephalopathy.

- Stroke recrudescence – reappearance or worsening of pre-existing stroke deficit usually due to toxic or metabolic factors (infection, sedative drugs, etc.).

■ Clinical Approach to a Patient With Suspected TIA

Evaluation of TIA is the same as for ischemic stroke, since the pathophysiology of TIA and ischemic stroke is the same. TIA should be thought of as a briefer, smaller ischemic stroke, but with the same implications for recurrence.

HISTORY AND PHYSICAL EXAM

- Make sure that the neurological symptoms have resolved!
  - If you document a normal neurological exam and later the patient develops recurrent neurological deficits, they can still be treated with tPA because the clock starts over from the time of new symptoms, as long as the patient was completely back to normal in between.
- Since you are likely to be seeing the patient after, and not during, the TIA, get an objective description as much as possible, perhaps from a witness:
  - "Were you able to move your arm?"
  - "Was his speech slurred?"
  - "Was she able to walk normally?"

BRAIN IMAGING

- Consider skipping CT and going straight to MRI and MRA if possible.

- Because of the proven benefit of CEA and stenting (see Chapter 8), careful vascular imaging with CTA or MRA is essential.
- CT is expected to be normal – because (a) it was transient ischemia; or (b) ischemia continues to be present but it's too small to see on CT; or (c) it was not ischemia.
- MRI is more likely than CT to be helpful – because (a) it shows you a small stroke that you didn't see on CT in about 50% of patients (ischemia improved to make the patient symptomatically back to baseline but tissue was damaged); or (b) it shows you a vascular lesion that, by association, makes you suspect that it was an ischemic event (small-vessel disease, old stroke, arterial stenosis, etc.); or (c) it shows you some other explanation of the transient event (subdural hematoma, tumor, etc.).

DECIDE WHETHER THIS IS MORE LIKELY A TIA OR SOMETHING ELSE

Other tests might be done to exclude non-TIA diagnoses if they are suspected.

- Electrocardiogram (ECG) is helpful because if you see atrial fibrillation, it was likely to have been a cardioembolic TIA. In these cases, initiating treatment with anticoagulation may prevent a stroke.
- Measurement of blood sugar is helpful because hypoglycemia can explain the event.
- Measurement of other electrolytes is helpful because electrolyte abnormalities may also explain the event.

MANAGEMENT

Again, the management is similar to that for acute ischemic stroke, as are the preventive measures.

- Observe the patient for 24 hours. Remember, if a patient develops new neurological symptoms he or she could be a candidate for tPA if no other exclusions exist.
- Start antiplatelets (consider dual antiplatelet therapy for 21 days) and consider starting a lipid-lowering agent.
- MRI to evaluate for new and old stroke.
- Carotid ultrasound and TCD, MRA of neck and brain, or CT angiogram of neck and brain to look for arterial stenosis. Be sure to evaluate the entire cerebrovascular system.
- ECG, and consider ECG telemetry, Holter monitor, or 30-day event monitor.
- Cardiovascular risk-factor evaluation of blood pressure, lipids, and fasting glucose.
- Consider echocardiogram for evaluation of cardioembolic source.
- Educate the patient about:
  - stroke risk factors, including hypertension, smoking, sedentary lifestyle, obesity, alcohol
  - medications prescribed for prevention
  - stroke symptoms to look for
  - emergency services for acute stroke symptoms
  - follow-up care after discharge from hospital

■ Prognosis After TIA

- After an ED visit for TIA:[2]
  - 5.3% stroke risk within 2 days
  - 10.5% stroke in 90 days (21% fatal, 64% disabling)
- 1 in 9 patients will have a stroke within 3 months.
- The key problem is trying to predict who will have a stroke (Tables 9.1 and 9.2).

Table 9.1 Risk stratification for stroke after TIA: the ABCD^2 score

Age	> 60 years	1 point
Blood pressure	> 140 mmHg systolic or > 90 mmHg diastolic at presentation	1 point
Clinical feature	Unilateral weakness	2 points
	Speech impairment in absence of unilateral weakness	1 point
Duration of symptoms	< 10 minutes	0 point
	10–59 minutes	1 point
	≥ 60 minutes	2 points
Diabetes		1 point
Total		**0–7 points**

Source: Johnston SC, Rothwell PM, Nguyen-Huynh MN, *et al.* Validation and refinement of scores to predict very early stroke risk after transient ischaemic attack. *Lancet* 2007; 369: 283–292.[3] Reproduced with permission.

Table 9.2 Stroke risk associated with ABCD^2 score

ABCD^2 score	Very low: 0–1 points	Low: 2–3 points	Moderate: 4–5 points	High: 6–7 points	All TIAs
Stroke within 2 days	0.0%	1.2%	4.1%	8.1%	3.9%
Stroke within 7 days	0.0%	1.4%	5.9%	11.7%	5.5%
Stroke within 90 days	1.7%	3.3%	9.8%	17.8%	9.2%

Adapted from: Johnston SC, Rothwell PM, Nguyen-Huynh MN, *et al.* Validation and refinement of scores to predict very early stroke risk after transient ischaemic attack. *Lancet* 2007; 369: 283–292.[3] Reproduced with permission.

References

1. Albers GW, Caplan LR, Easton JD, *et al.* Transient ischemic attack: proposal for a new definition. *N Engl J Med* 2002; 347: 1713–1716.
2. Johnston SC, Gress DR, Browner WS, Sidney S. Short-term prognosis after emergency department diagnosis of TIA. *JAMA* 2000; 284: 2901–2906.
3. Johnston SC, Rothwell PM, Nguyen-Huynh MN, *et al.* Validation and refinement of scores to predict very early stroke risk after transient ischaemic attack. *Lancet* 2007; 369: 283–292.

10

Less Common Causes of Stroke

Most strokes are caused by the mechanisms already described, i.e., cardioembolism, atherosclerosis, and small-vessel disease, but at least 20% are due to other mechanisms. This is even more likely in younger patients (< 40 years old), and in older patients without atherosclerotic risk factors. The following is our approach to stroke diagnosis in younger patients and older patients in whom the cause remains obscure after the usual evaluation of the heart for sources of emboli and cerebral vessels for atherosclerosis, or who continue to have strokes despite standard treatment with antithrombotic agents and control of risk factors.

■ Causes

EXTRACRANIAL CAUSES

1. **Arterial dissection** (carotid, vertebral, aortic) – see Chapter 8
   - Can be traumatic or spontaneous.
   - Inquire about personal or family history of arterial dissections (can be in other vessels in the body such as aortic or renal arteries), collagen vascular diseases (such as Ehlers–Danlos type 4 or Marfan syndrome).

- Ask about any recent blunt trauma to head or neck, chiropractic manipulation of the neck, or sudden occupational/accidental movements of the head/neck.

2. **Aortic arch atheroma or unstable non-stenotic carotid plaque**
   - Vessel or cardiac imaging should always include the aortic arch.
   - Higher-grade aortic atheromas (grades 3–5) are associated with increased risk of strokes. Grading is based on plaque thickness and sessile versus mobile nature of the plaque.
   - Some carotid bifurcation plaques causing < 60% stenosis can still embolize. How to identify and manage them is still uncertain.

3. **Paradoxical embolus of venous clot** through a patent foramen ovale (PFO) or pulmonary arteriovenous malformation (AVM) – see Chapter 8
   - Echocardiogram or TCD ordered with bubble study help make the diagnosis.
   - Association of a PFO with an atrial septal aneurysm may increase the risk of initial or recurrent strokes, but this is still debated.
   - Larger PFO size and larger right-to-left shunts may also increase the stroke risk.
   - Pulmonary AVMs are best visualized on a CT of the chest with contrast.

4. **Air embolism**
   - Uncommon but can be fatal.
   - Usually occurs iatrogenically as a result of central venous catheter placement, surgical procedures, ventilator-induced barotrauma, decompression sickness, or aorto-esophageal fistula.
   - In the acute setting, multiple hypodensities can be seen in the parenchyma and intracranial vessels on non-contrast head CT.
   - There is an increased trend towards treating air embolism with hyperbaric chambers in capable centers.

5. **Fibromuscular dysplasia (FMD)** of extracranial carotid artery
   - More common in middle-aged women with hypertension.

- Can lead to embolism if associated with aneurysm or web formation.
- Treatment includes antiplatelets, anticoagulation, or less commonly endovascular stenting or vascular surgery.

INTRACRANIAL CAUSES

1. **Cerebral venous sinus thrombosis** – discussed in Chapter 11
2. **Vasculitides** (giant cell arteritis, primary CNS angiitis, polyarteritis nodosa, Takayasu aortitis, other collagen vascular diseases)
   - Commonly associated with insidious headaches.
   - Relapsing in nature, with imaging revealing strokes of different ages.
   - Vascular imaging may reveal beading of distal intracranial vessels.
   - CSF analysis usually has an inflammatory profile.
   - Treatment is with antiplatelets, steroids, and long-term immunosuppressive therapies.
3. **Infection-related vasculopathies** (e.g., HIV, VZV)
4. **Moyamoya**
   - "Puff of smoke" in Japanese, for the classic appearance produced by the brittle collaterals found on conventional angiogram.
   - Refers to the progressive narrowing of the terminal ICAs and proximal branches of the arteries making up the circle of Willis.
   - Affects Asian populations predominantly, and women more than men.
   - Moyamoya syndrome (as opposed to moyamoya disease) is associated with predisposing conditions such as NF-1, SLE, Down syndrome, or sickle cell disease. It is important to test for these conditions in a patient with suspected moyamoya. Advanced atherosclerosis can also lead to a moyamoya syndrome.
   - Treatment usually includes antiplatelets and, in advanced cases, superficial temporal artery (STA)–MCA bypass or revascularization procedures based on angiogenesis such as encephalo-duro-arterio-

synangiosis (EDAS) or encephalo-duro-arterio-myo-synangiosis (EDAMS).

5. **Intravascular lymphoma**
6. **Reversible cerebral vasoconstriction syndrome (RCVS)**
   - Classically associated with thunderclap headaches.
   - Risk factors include pregnancy or postpartum, use of sympathomimetics, immunosuppressants (e.g., FK508, cyclophosphamide), SSRIs, triptans or ergotamines.
   - May see beading of vessels during attack.
   - Usually a monophasic course.
   - CSF is often normal.
   - Treatment includes calcium channel blockers such as nimodipine or verapamil (given IV, PO, or IA), IV magnesium. There is no definitive role for steroids.
   - Prognosis is excellent.

HEMATOLOGICAL CAUSES

1. **Hypercoagulability** – inherited or acquired. if no primary hematological problem is evident, look for underlying cancer.
2. **Sickle cell disease** – can lead to strokes as a result of vaso-occlusive crises. Can also produce a moyamoya syndrome over time. Twenty-five percent of patients with sickle cell disease will have a stroke before the age of 45. Recurrence rate is very high if not treated. Standard of care is chronic transfusion therapy in patients with peak systolic velocities > 200 cm/s on TCD. Annual TCD screening is important in children from age 2 to 16 years. More frequent screening is recommended for symptomatic patients. In the STOP study, the goal of transfusion therapy was to achieve a hemoglobin-S fraction of less than 30%, which resulted in a 92% reduction in stroke risk compared to the standard-care group.[1]

3. **Thrombotic microangiopathies**(thrombotic thrombocytopenic purpura, TTP; disseminated intravascular coagulation, DIC) – TTP complicated by stroke should be treated with urgent plasmapheresis.

GENETIC CAUSES

1. **CADASIL** (cerebral autosomal dominant arteriopathy with subcortical infarcts and leukoencephalopathy)
   - Age of onset 40–50s.
   - *NOTCH3* gene mutation.
   - Migraines are common. Progresses to pseudobulbar affect and dementia.
   - Radiographic findings: (1) confluent white-matter hyperintensities (leukoaraiosis) in subcortical/periventricular areas, (2) multiple lacunar infarcts in deep gray matter, and (3) microbleeds. White-matter changes tend to have a predilection for the external capsules and anterior temporal lobes.
   - Skin biopsy is easy and diagnostic.
   - Genetic analysis is the gold standard but is expensive.
2. **CARASIL** (cerebral autosomal recessive arteriopathy with subcortical infarcts and leukoencephalopathy)
   - Very rare.
   - Age of onset 20–30s.
   - *HTRA1* gene mutation.
   - More severe than CADASIL.
   - Associated with premature alopecia, progressive dementia, and lumbar spondylosis.
   - Subcortical white-matter hyperintensities with leukoaraiosis and lacunar infarcts in deep gray matter but no microbleeds.

3. **MELAS** (mitochondrial encephalomyopathy, lactic acidosis, and stroke-like episodes)
   - A mitochondrial maternally inherited disorder, due to an A3243G mutation in the gene encoding tRNA.
   - Characterized by:
     - recurrent strokes before age 40
     - encephalopathy, progressive cognitive delay, seizures
     - acidosis, emesis, abdominal pains, myopathy
     - sensorineural hearing loss, cataracts
     - short stature
   - Diagnosis is via genetic testing. Imaging shows cortical strokes of different ages, mostly in the parietal–temporal and parietal–occipital areas.
   - No specific treatment exists. However, a few agents have been used, such as L-arginine, L-citrulline during attacks and during the interictal phase (nitric oxide precursors increase availability of nitric oxide, cerebral vasodilation, and cerebral perfusion), levocarnitine, and coenzyme Q10. Valproate use is discouraged, as it can paradoxically increase seizure frequency, and statins can result in worsening of the myopathy.

4. **Fabry disease**
   - X-linked lysosomal storage disease.
   - Alpha-galactosidase-A deficiency.
   - Associated with angiokeratomas and painful neuropathy.
   - Enzyme replacement is now available.

DRUG-RELATED CAUSES

Sympathomimetic drugs are not an uncommon etiology of stroke in the young population. Amphetamines and cocaine can cause strokes due to hypertensive crisis, arterial dissection, vasospasm, or vasculitis.

■ Tests to Consider

1. **Urine drug screen**
2. **Check medications and supplements that the patient is taking at home**
3. **Hypercoagulable states –** There is no consensus on when to test for these, but it should certainly be done if there is a positive family history of clotting or previous history of DVT, pulmonary embolism, or miscarriage.

   Arterial thromboses
   - Antiphospholipid antibody panel
     - Anticardiolipin IgM and IgG
     - Beta-2 glycoprotein IgM and IgG (not to be confused with beta-2 microglobulin)
     - Lupus anticoagulant (testing can be both mixing and Russell viper venom test)
   - Hemoglobin electrophoresis
   - Homocysteine level

   Venous thromboses – same as above, plus:
   - Protein C
   - Protein S
   - Antithrombin III
   - Activated protein C (APC) resistance (biochemical test for factor V Leiden, so you don't need the DNA test if you order this)
   - Factor V Leiden – DNA test
   - Factor II (prothrombin gene) G20210A – DNA test
   - Protein C, S, and antithrombin III can be falsely elevated acutely in stroke patients

4. **Autoimmune laboratory testing**
   - ESR, high-sensitivity CRP (hsCRP)
   - ANA, anti-dsDNA, anti-Smith, anti-RNP, C3, C4
   - SS-A, SS-B
   - c-ANCA, p-ANCA

5. **Fibrinogen, PT, INR, PTT**
6. **CT chest/abdomen/pelvis with contrast**
   - To evaluate for occult malignancy as cause of hypercoagulable state associated with stroke
   - To evaluate for pulmonary AVM as a source of embolism
7. **Pelvic MRV and lower-extremity Doppler**
   - If considering paradoxical embolism of venous clot through PFO or pulmonary AVM
8. **Conventional angiogram**
   - To evaluate for fibromuscular dysplasia, RCVS, vasculitis
9. **Lumbar puncture**
   - To evaluate for infections associated with stroke (HIV, VZV), vasculitis
10. **Genetic testing**
   - Recommend genetic counseling
   - CADASIL: *NOTCH3* gene mutation
   - CARASIL: *HTRA1* gene mutation
   - Fabry disease: alpha-galactosidase-A enzyme testing
   - MELAS: mitochondrial DNA mutation of *MT-TL1* or *MT-ND5*

References

1. Adams R, McKie V, Hsu L, *et al.* Prevention of a first stroke by transfusion in children with abnormal results of transcranial Doppler ultrasonography. *N Engl J Med* 1998; 339: 5–11.

11

Cerebral Venous Sinus Thrombosis

■ Epidemiology

Cerebral venous sinus thrombosis (CVST) is the thrombosis of dural venous sinuses and/or cerebral veins. It accounts for 0.5% of all strokes. It occurs predominantly in the younger population (usually < 50 years old, median age of 37). Female-to-male ratio is 3 to 1, likely secondary to sex-specific thrombogenic states including pregnancy, puerperium, oral contraceptive pill use, and hormonal therapy.[1]

■ Pathogenesis

Venous thrombosis can cause localized edema and infarction.
Thrombosis of major sinuses or the deep venous system (Figure 11.1) can lead to global edema and intracranial hypertension due to the impairment of CSF drainage.

■ Risk Factors[3]

- At least one risk factor is detected in 85% of cases.
- Transient risk factors include pregnancy, puerperium, infections (e.g., meningitis, sinusitis, mastoiditis, otitis media), procedure (e.g.,

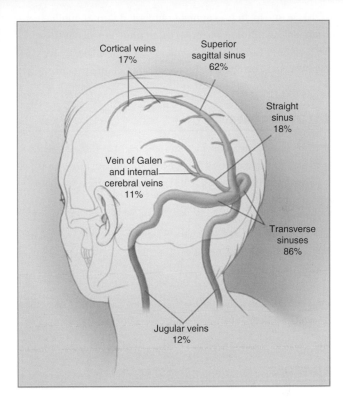

Figure 11.1 Frequency of cerebral venous thrombosis by site. (A black and white version of this figure will appear in some formats. For the color version, please refer to the plate section.)

Adapted from: Stam J. Thrombosis of the cerebral veins and sinuses. *N Engl J Med* 2005; 352: 1791–1798.[2]

intracranial surgery, lumbar puncture), dehydration, exposure to drugs, and head trauma.

• CVST can also occur in association with cancer, and may develop before the cancer is diagnosed.

- Chronic risk factors include acquired or inherited thrombophilia (e.g., antiphospholipid syndrome, factor V Leiden mutation, factor II mutation (prothrombin G20210A), protein C/S deficiencies).
- Multiple risk factors are commonly encountered in one patient.

■ Clinical Picture

Headache is the most common symptom (80–90% of cases) and, when isolated, can lead to the diagnosis being overlooked. Four clinical syndromes are frequently seen with CVST, and these can be found in isolation or combined:[4,5]

1. seizures (40%)
2. intracranial hypertension (e.g., headache, altered sensorium, diplopia, papilledema, bilateral sixth nerve palsies) (37%)
3. focal neurological deficit (20–37%)
4. encephalopathy (20–30 %)

Hemorrhagic conversion of a venous infarct occurs in up to 40% of cases. It has been associated with older age, female sex, and acute onset.

■ Diagnosis

- A high level of suspicion is needed to make the correct diagnosis. Imaging is crucial. Clues to diagnosis on initial imaging include bilateral paramedian hypodensities, infarction that does not respect an arterial territory, or parenchymal hemorrhage in an unusual location adjacent to a venous sinus.[6,7]
- The preferred neuroimaging modality is MRI and MR venography (MRV). The SWI sequence of the MRI allows identification of isolated cortical venous thrombosis. Contrast MRV is more sensitive than time-of-flight MRV.

- CT and CT venography (CTV) can also be used but are not as sensitive as MRI. On CT head, a "dense cord" sign might be seen (hyperdense thrombosed vein or sinus). An "empty delta" sign can be seen on contrast CT. CTV is not sensitive enough to detect cortical vein thromboses.
- Conventional angiography is rarely used unless non-invasive imaging is equivocal or it is needed for therapeutic intervention. Also, the altered venous drainage associated with CVST can result in a chronic dural fistula, which can only be diagnosed by arteriography including the external carotid and vertebral arteries.

■ Acute Management

- **Anticoagulation** – Initial systemic anticoagulation using either unfractionated heparin (UFH) or low-molecular-weight heparin (LMWH) is the mainstay of therapy, despite the limited evidence coming from two small randomized studies.[8,9] In one study, LMWH was seen to be more efficacious (better functional outcome at 6 months) and perhaps safer (less risk of ICH) than UFH. It is recommended to anticoagulate even in the face of hemorrhagic transformation or venous-related ICH. The purpose of anticoagulation is to prevent extension of the thrombus and facilitate recanalization.
- **Osmotherapy** – Osmotherapy can be very effective in reducing vasogenic edema secondary to venous obstruction. It should be started as soon as edema begins to produce mass effect on adjacent structures (see Chapter 7).
- **Endovascular therapy** – Intra-arterial thrombolysis and mechanical thrombectomy (using stent retrievers, aspiration devices, or balloon venoplasty) have been used but efficacy has not been established because of the lack of randomized trials.[10,11] Endovascular therapy is

used when systemic anticoagulation is unsuccessful at recanalization and the patient's neurological status is deteriorating.

- **Decompressive hemicraniectomy** – Very limited data exist on this therapy. It remains an option for patients who develop refractory intracranial hypertension related to malignant hemispheric edema/infarction.[12] The potential for expansion of the intracranial hemorrhage is a worrisome complication of the surgery.

■ Chronic Management

The duration for anticoagulation usually takes into account recurrences, provoked versus unprovoked CVST, bleeding risk, and patient preference. It is recommended to treat provoked CVST with 3–6 months of warfarin after the provoking stimulus is rectified, aiming for a target INR of 2.0–3.0. Unprovoked CVSTs are usually treated with warfarin for 6–12 months. Recurrent CVSTs or those caused by an underlying thrombophilia may require lifelong anticoagulation. These recommendations are based on consensus rather than a strong evidence base.[1]

■ Complications of CVST

- **Seizures** – more common in cases of intracranial hypertension, venous infarction, or hemorrhagic conversion. No prophylaxis is recommended, but seizures should be treated.
- **Hydrocephalus** – resulting from obstruction of CSF drainage at the arachnoid granulation level. May warrant the placement of a ventriculostomy or a shunt.
- **Intracranial hypertension** – see Chapter 12.

■ Prognosis and Recurrence

Women tend to have a better prognosis than men (in one study, 81% versus 71% fully recovered).[13] The recurrence risk of CVST is usually low. About 2.2% of patients with CVST had recurrences within 18 months in a multicenter observational study.[14] The incidence of any VTE (not just CVST) is 6.5% per year. Some inherited thrombophilias are considered mild in that the risk of recurrent VTE is lower (11% at 5 years). These include heterozygous factor V Leiden, heterozygous prothrombin G20210A mutations, dysfibrinogenemia, and elevated factor VIII. The severe thrombophilias, such as protein C/S, and antithrombin III deficiencies, antiphospholipid antibodies, and homozygous factor V Leiden or prothrombin G20210A mutation are associated with a higher recurrence risk of VTE (40% at 5 years).[15]

References

1. Saposnik G, Barinagarrementeria F, Brown R, *et al.* Diagnosis and management of cerebral venous thrombosis: a statement for healthcare professionals from the American Heart Association/American Stroke Association. *Stroke* 2011; 42: 1158–1192.

2. Stam J. Thrombosis of the cerebral veins and sinuses. *N Engl J Med* 2005; 352: 1791–1798.

3. Bousser MG, Ferro JM. Cerebral venous thrombosis: an update. *Lancet Neurol* 2007; 6: 162–170.

4. Biousse V, Ameri A, Bousser MG. Isolated intracranial hypertension as the only sign of cerebral venous thrombosis. *Neurology* 1999; 53: 1537–1542.

5. Luo Y, Tian X, Wang X. Diagnosis and treatment of cerebral venous thrombosis: a review. *Front Aging Neurosci* 2018; 10: 2.

6. Wasay M, Azeemuddin M. Neuroimaging of cerebral venous thrombosis. *J Neuroimaging* 2005; 15: 118–128.

7. Ganeshan D, Narlawar R, McCann C, *et al.* Cerebral venous thrombosis—a pictorial review. *Eur J Radiol* 2010; 74: 110–116.

8. Einhaupl KM, Villringer A, Meister W, *et al.* Heparin treatment in sinus venous thrombosis. *Lancet* 1991; 338: 597–600.

9. Coutinho JM, Ferro JM, Canhao P, *et al.* Unfractionated or low-molecular-weight heparin for the treatment of cerebral venous thrombosis. *Stroke* 2010; 41: 2575–2580.

10. Stolz E, Trittmacher S, Rahimi A, *et al.* Influence of recanalization on outcome in dural sinus thrombosis: a prospective study. *Stroke* 2004; 35: 544–547.

11. Borhani Haghighi A, Mahmoodi M, Edgell RC, *et al.* Mechanical thrombectomy for cerebral venous sinus thrombosis: a comprehensive literature review. *Clin Appl Thromb Hemost* 2014; 20: 507–512.

12. Zuurbier SM, Coutinho JM, Majoie CB, *et al.* Decompressive hemicraniectomy in severe cerebral venous thrombosis: a prospective case series. *J Neurol* 2012; 259: 1099–1105.

13. Coutinho JM, Ferro JM, Canhao P, *et al.* Cerebral venous and sinus thrombosis in women. *Stroke* 2009; 40: 2356–2361.

14. Ferro J, Canhao P, Stam J, *et al.* Prognosis of cerebral vein and dural sinus thrombosis: results of the International Study on Cerebral Vein and Dural Sinus Thrombosis (ISCVT). *Stroke* 2004; 35: 664–670

15. Martinelli I, Bucciarelli P, Passamonti SM, *et al.* Long-term evaluation of the risk of recurrence after cerebral sinus-venous thrombosis. *Circulation* 2010; 121: 2740–2746.

12

Intracerebral Hemorrhage

In this chapter, we consider spontaneous hemorrhage into the brain parenchyma and ventricles (intracerebral hemorrhage, ICH). Non-traumatic bleeding into the subarachnoid space (subarachnoid hemorrhage, SAH) is covered in Chapter 13. Traumatic subdural and epidural hemorrhages are not covered in this book.

Intracerebral hemorrhage is associated with very high morbidity and mortality. It is important to realize that, as with acute ischemic strokes, time is of the essence in ICH. The reason for this is that the blood accumulates rapidly, and the volume of the hematoma is the most important determinant of outcome.[1] As a result of bleeding, there can be rapid development of intracranial hypertension as a result of mass effect from the blood, and occasional hydrocephalus in cases of intraventricular hemorrhage (IVH). Therefore, anything that can be done in the first few minutes after the onset of ICH to limit bleeding will reduce morbidity. In the last decade, progress has been made in the pharmacological reversal of coagulopathy and "optimal" blood-pressure management after ICH. These are discussed extensively later in the chapter. In the days to weeks following the ictus, vasogenic edema develops around the hematoma and can contribute to significant (and sometimes life-threatening) mass effect, especially in large ICH or those associated with an inflammatory or vascular etiology (e.g., tumors, vascular malformations). We address medical and surgical management to combat brain swelling and its consequences in Chapter 7.

■ Definition

Intracerebral hemorrhage is spontaneous bleeding into the brain parenchyma or ventricles from a ruptured artery, vein, or other vascular structure (Figure 12.1). It is important to distinguish primary ICH, which is the topic of this chapter, from hemorrhagic transformation of an ischemic infarct, covered in

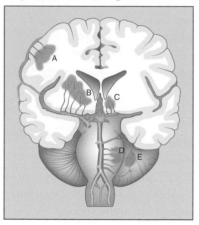

Figure 12.1 Location of hemorrhages: (A) penetrating cortical branches of the anterior, middle, or posterior cerebral arteries; (B) basal ganglia, originating from ascending lenticulostriate branches of the middle cerebral artery; (C) the thalamus, originating from ascending thalamogeniculate branches of the posterior cerebral artery; (D) the pons, originating from paramedian branches of the basilar artery; and (E) the cerebellum, originating from penetrating branches of the posterior inferior, anterior inferior, or superior cerebellar arteries. (A black and white version of this figure will appear in some formats. For the color version, please refer to the plate section.)
Source: Qureshi AI, Tuhrim S, Broderick JP, *et al.* Spontaneous intracerebral hemorrhage. *N Engl J Med* 2001; 344: 1450–1460.[2] Copyright © 2001 Massachusetts Medical Society. Reproduced with permission from the Massachusetts Medical Society.

Chapter 7. In primary ICH, the initial event is vascular rupture, while in hemorrhagic transformation the initial event is vascular occlusion. This is obviously an important distinction, since the etiologies and treatments are completely different. The term "hemorrhagic stroke" is used loosely and imprecisely and is often applied to either of these conditions. We prefer the more precise distinction.

■ Etiology

1. **Hypertension**
   (most common) – classic locations for hypertensive intracerebral hemorrhage:
   - Basal ganglia (putamen most common)
   - Thalamus
   - Pons
   - Cerebellum
2. **Cerebral amyloid angiopathy**
   - Results from beta-amyloid protein deposition in the walls of small and mid-sized arteries, compromising vessel wall integrity.
   - More often cortical in location than hypertensive hemorrhages.
   - Older patients (> 65 years) or positive family history.
   - Frequently associated with cognitive impairment or dementia.
   - Microbleeds in cortical locations seen as hypointense/black lesions (due to hemosiderin deposition) on gradient-echo (GRE) or susceptibility-weighted imaging (SWI) sequences on MRI.
3. **Other angiopathies** – moyamoya, vasculitides, RCVS
4. **Drugs**
   - Iatrogenic, e.g., heparin or warfarin
   - Drugs of abuse, especially cocaine
5. **Vascular malformation** – aneurysm, AVM, cavernous malformation

6. **Cerebral vein thrombosis** (see Chapter 11)
   - Caused by bleeding from congested vein feeding into an occluded cortical vein or venous sinus thrombosis.
   - Technically considered transformation of a "venous infarct."
   - The clinical presentation of the thrombosis may be dominated by the development of ICH. This is different from arterial occlusion with hemorrhagic transformation, where the initial clinical presentation is almost always the result of the infarct, and the hemorrhage comes hours later.

7. **Tumor**
   - Primary tumors (e.g., glioblastoma, pilocytic astrocytoma)
   - Metastatic tumors (e.g., melanoma, breast carcinoma, papillary carcinoma of thyroid)

8. **Trauma**
   - Closed head injury
   - Penetrating injury
   - Explosive blast injury

9. **Coagulopathy**
   - Liver cirrhosis
   - Disseminated intravascular coagulation (DIC)

■ Presentation

- You cannot distinguish ICH from ischemic stroke on the basis of the clinical presentation – they may look exactly alike. This is the reason brain imaging is so critical in initial stroke management, since brain bleeding can be readily detected by CT or MRI immediately after it occurs.
- Clinical features that might suggest ICH rather than an infarct include headache, accelerated hypertension, vomiting (always a bad sign in an acute stroke patient, usually indicative of increasing ICP), decreasing level of consciousness, or a dilated and fixed pupil.

■ Diagnosis and Evaluation

As with ischemic stroke, management in the first few hours may make the difference between a good and bad outcome. We recommend the following initial assessment.

1. **History and physical exam**
   - Look for signs of trauma.
   - Glasgow Coma Scale (GCS) and brainstem reflexes if comatose, NIHSS score if awake.
   - Consider intubation for airway protection.
   - Measure blood pressure (see subsequent comment for details on blood-pressure management).

2. **Non-contrast CT**
   - This is the gold-standard test to diagnose an ICH in the hyperacute/ acute phase.
   - Repeat the CT if patient was transferred from outside hospital (the bleed could have extended en route).
     - Would repeat in 6–24 hours to gauge stability of the bleed.
     - Repeat STAT in case of neurological deterioration.
   - Where did the bleed start?
   - Is there significant mass effect, intraventricular hemorrhage (IVH), or hydrocephalus?
   - Measure the volume: (diameter A × diameter B × C)/2. (A and B = perpendicular diameters of the hematoma on the CT slice with the largest area of parenchymal hemorrhage, C = number of slices that show hemorrhage × thickness of the slice) (Figure 12.2).

3. **Check platelet count, INR, and PTT, and urine drug screen**

4. **ECG**: abnormalities may point to MI or stress cardiomyopathy. In case of abnormality, obtain cardiac enzymes.

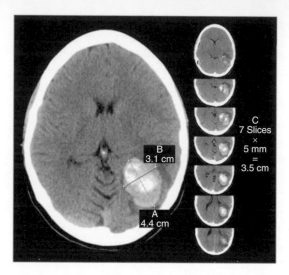

Figure 12.2 Calculating ICH volume on a CT image.
Source: Beslow LA, Ichord RN, Kasner SE, *et al.* ABC/XYZ estimates intracerebral hemorrhage volume as a percent of total brain volume in children. *Stroke* 2010; 41: 691–694.[3] Reproduced with permission.

5. **Consider vascular imaging study**

   (MRA, CTA, or DSA) to rule out AVM, dural AV fistula, or aneurysm, especially if:

   - younger patient

     or

   - significant SAH is present

     or

   - ICH is in an atypical lobar or cortical location, or has some other atypical appearance.

6. **Consider MRI** (not urgent):

   - To look for multiple old hemorrhages or microbleeds that might suggest amyloid angiopathy. Requires GRE or SWI sequences.

- To exclude underlying tumor (this is rather rare and usually requires follow-up imaging in 6–8 weeks after most of the blood has been reabsorbed). Requires gadolinium to look for enhancement indicative of blood–brain barrier disruption.
- To check for venous thrombosis, order MR venogram if the suspicion is high: hemorrhage high in convexity, bilateral paramedian in cases of deep venous system thrombosis, substantial perihematomal edema, or temporal lobe hemorrhage without trauma.

7. **Consider getting a neurosurgery consult**
   (see *Surgical Intervention*, below):
   - For possible hematoma evacuation or ventriculostomy.
   - If aneurysm or AVM suspected.

■ Management

It is important to talk with family and start the process of coming to terms with the often poor prognosis (see *Prognosis and Outcome*, below). This is a very important management consideration. Discuss "do not resuscitate" (DNR) issues. However, on the first day, don't be too certain of bad outcome unless herniation has already occurred and the brainstem is significantly compromised. Comatose patients can wake up, especially if the mass effect is decompressed spontaneously into the ventricle, or by surgical intervention. Do not withdraw support in the ED.

HEMATOMA ENLARGEMENT TREATMENT

Hematoma enlargement occurs in 20–35% of ICH.[4]
- All locations.

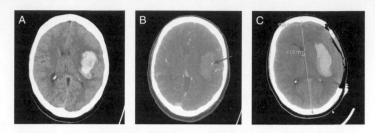

Figure 12.3 Hematoma expansion and CT spot sign. (A) Initial non-contrast head CT showing a left basal ganglia ICH measuring 47 mL. (B) A single spot sign (area of active contrast extravasation, *arrow*) seen within the ICH on CT angiography. (C) No significant expansion of the ICH (volume 55 mL) on a follow-up CT 7 hours later, attesting to the fact that the accuracy of the spot sign as a radiographic predictor of hematoma expansion may be lower than initially believed. (N.B. This patient had decompressive hemicraniectomy in the interim, but no hematoma evacuation or aspiration.)

Source: Brouwers HB and Greenberg SM. Hematoma expansion following acute intracerebral hemorrhage. *Cerebrovasc Dis* 2013; 35: 195–201. Reproduced with permission

- Usually in the first few hours after onset of symptoms, but almost always in the first 24 hours.
- May occur later in patients with coagulopathy.
- Associated with much worse prognosis.
- Independent radiographic predictors of hematoma expansion are numerous and include:[5]
  - Large initial hematoma volume.
  - Hematoma heterogeneity – swirl sign, blend sign, island sign, presence of a fluid level.
  - Active extravasation – spot sign and leak sign. The spot sign is one of the most studied predictor signs of hematoma expansion. While it was thought to be a radiographic sign with good sensitivity and specificity, a preplanned study nested within the multicenter trial ATACH-2 (see below) has more recently shown that the sensitivity and specificity of the spot sign were only 54%

and 63% respectively, making it not as accurate a tool for hematoma expansion prediction (Figure 12.3).[6]

1. Aggressive Blood-Pressure Reduction

- BP elevation is associated with hematoma expansion, poor functional outcome, and higher mortality.
- Lowering SBP to 140 mmHg is safe (no significant perihematomal ischemia) and is recommended in the latest guidelines.[7]
- See below for more detailed information on BP management in acute ICH.

2. Activated Factor VII

- In the FAST trial, activated factor VII (NovoSeven) was found to reduce hematoma expansion but did not have any effect on survival or functional outcome at 90 days. Possible explanations are that it was given too late (on average 4 hours after symptom onset) or in patients whose hematomas were already so large that they were in any case doomed to poor outcome.[8]
- Activated factor VII is expensive and can have dose-related occlusive complications such as stroke, myocardial infarction, pulmonary embolism, etc.
- Patients with associated arterial occlusive diseases (coronary or cerebral ischemia, peripheral vascular disease, or pulmonary embolism), or who have already herniated, are not considered.
- Further study is needed before it is used routinely.

COAGULOPATHY REVERSAL

1. Vitamin K Antagonist (VKA)-Related Intracerebral Hemorrhage

- **Goal:** normal INR using prothrombin complex concentrates (PCC) or fresh frozen plasma (FFP) *and* vitamin K.

- **Obtain non-contrast CT immediately**
  a. Labs: INR, PTT, thrombin time, D-dimers, fibrinogen, CBC, type and crossmatch
  b. Vitamin K 10 mg IV over 10 minutes (repeat daily for 3 days) should always be given, because it maintains the reversal over time:
     - Slow onset (2 hours)
     - Effect peaks at 24 hours if hepatic function not impaired
- **PCC versus FFP**
  a. Three different formulations:
     - Three-factor PCC: II, IX, and X
     - Four-factor PCC: II, VII, IX, and X
     - Activated PCC (aPCC): four coagulation factors. Example: FEIBA (Factor Eight Inhibitor Bypassing Activity)
  b. Dosing of PCC: 25–50 IU/kg, depending on patient's weight, INR, and the preparation
  c. Advantages of PCC over FFP:
     - Faster administration (25 minutes versus 30–120 minutes)
     - No need to thaw
     - No need for type and crossmatch
     - Lower risk of infections and transfusion reactions
     - Much smaller volume than FFP (~250 mL/unit FFP) – important in patients with or at risk for pulmonary edema
  d. Advantages of FFP over PCC:
     - Far less expensive
     - More widely available
  e. The recently published INCH trial compared PCC to FFP in reversing warfarin-induced ICH:[9]
     - PCC achieved faster and more complete INR normalization (≤ 1.2 within 3 hours).
     - PCC was associated with less hematoma growth, but there was no difference in functional outcome or mortality at 90 days.

- Other studies of PCC versus FFP in non-brain bleeding have shown lower mortality with PCC.

2. DOAC-Related Intracerebral Hemorrhage

The direct oral anticoagulants, apixaban, edoxaban, dabigatran, and rivaroxaban, are being increasingly prescribed because of their easier use, equal or higher efficacy, and usually better safety profile compared with vitamin K antagonists. As a result of this increased utilization, we are seeing more DOAC-related ICH.

- **Specific antidotes**
  a. Direct thrombin inhibitor – dabigatran
    - Idarucizumab, a humanized monoclonal antibody fragment, is dabigatran's antidote and reverses completely the effect of the direct thrombin inhibitor within minutes. In the US, idarucizumab was approved by the FDA in 2015.
    - Dose: 5 g IV (two separate vials each containing 2.5 g/50 mL).
  b. Factor Xa inhibitors – apixaban, edoxaban, rivaroxaban
    - Andexanet alpha was approved by the FDA in May 2018. It is a decoy receptor specific for the factor Xa inhibitors and reverses their effect within 2 minutes.
    - Dose: 400 or 800 mg IV bolus followed by 4 or 8 mg/minute IV infusion for up to 120 minutes.
    - Regimen intensity depends on dose of the factor Xa inhibitor and timing since the last dose.

- **Non-specific reversals**
  a. Activated charcoal – largely replaced by idarucizumab but can be considered within 3–4 hours of ingestion of dabigatran. Acts by reducing gastrointestinal absorption of dabigatran. Not useful for factor Xa inhibitors.
  b. Hemodialysis – filters out the non-protein-bound fraction of dabigatran (two-thirds of the drug is unbound).

c. PCC – incompletely reverses the effect of factor Xa inhibitors.

d. Factor eight inhibitor bypassing agent (FEIBA) – has been used in cases of ICH secondary to factor Xa inhibitors or direct thrombin inhibitors.

3. Antiplatelet Agent-Related Intracerebral Hemorrhage

- **The PATCH trial** randomized patients who had used an antiplatelet agent (APA) within the last 7 days to either one platelet transfusion or standard care.[10]

  a. The intervention arm had higher odds of death or severe disability (mRS 4–6) at 3 months (OR 2.05, 95% CI 1.18–3.56).

  b. Platelet transfusion in the setting of APA-related ICH therefore cannot be recommended.

  c. Platelet transfusions are often still given to patients who require surgical decompression in the setting of APA use, although the data for this are limited.

- **Alternatives to platelet transfusions** in APA-related ICH:

  a. DDAVP (desmopressin) 0.3 µg/kg by slow IV infusion (also used in patients with von Willebrand disease and chronic kidney disease).

  b. Activated recombinant factor VII has also been used, but there is a risk of thrombosis and it is therefore not currently recommended.

  c. Antifibrinolytic drugs, such as tranexamic acid or aminocaproic acid, have been used, but there is little rationale for their use in this situation and there are no data demonstrating benefit.

4. Heparin- and Heparinoid-Related Intracerebral Hemorrhage

- **Unfractionated heparin**

  a. Within 30 minutes of heparin discontinuation: 1 mg protamine per 100 units of heparin infused in the last 2 hours.

   b. Within 30–60 minutes of heparin discontinuation: 0.5–0.75 mg
     protamine per 100 units of heparin infused in the last 2 hours.

   c. Maximum dose of protamine = 50 mg.

   d. Monitor PTT 15 minutes after dose and then in 2 hours. May repeat
     dose of protamine if PTT still elevated.

   e. Side effects of protamine include: flushing, hypotension, bradycardia,
     dyspnea, and pulmonary hypertension.

- **Low-molecular-weight heparin (LMWH)** – reversal with protamine is
  not complete (reverses ~60–75% of anti-Xa activity).

   a. Last dose ≤ 8 hours: 1 mg protamine per 1 mg of LMWH.

   b. Last dose > 8 hours: 0.5 mg protamine per 1 mg of LMWH.

   c. Maximum dose of protamine = 50 mg.

WHAT IS THE TARGET BLOOD PRESSURE AFTER ICH?

1. Does Lowering Blood Pressure Cause Ischemia or Reduce the Risk of Rebleeding?

- Several studies, such as the ICH ADAPT trial, have shown that acutely
  lowering the blood pressure does not lead to hypoperfusion and
  ischemia of the perihematomal zone and does not increase mortality or
  morbidity.[11]

- Target blood pressure – Two recent trials, INTERACT-2 and ATACH-2,
  have addressed blood-pressure targets after ICH. These trials compared
  two intensity levels of systolic BP reduction: < 140 mmHg (ATACH-2)
  and < 180 mmHg (INTERACT-2), usually employing intravenous
  nicardipine.[12,13]

- More intense BP reduction, below SBP 140 mmHg, had no effect on
  mortality, major disability, or reduction in hematoma expansion in the
  two trials (Figures 12.4 and 12.5).

- There was a significant improvement in functional outcome as
  measured by ordinal shift in mRS in INTERACT-2 but not in ATACH-2.

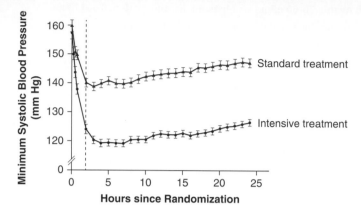

Figure 12.4 Minimum systolic blood pressure in the two treatment arms of the ATACH-2 trial during the first 24 hours post-randomization.

Source: ATACH-2 Trial Investigators, Neurological Emergency Treatment Trials Network. Intensive blood-pressure lowering in patients with acute cerebral hemorrhage. *N Engl J Med* 2016; 375: 1033–1043.[13] Copyright © 2016 Massachusetts Medical Society. Reproduced with permission from the Massachusetts Medical Society.

- There was also a higher incidence rate of acute kidney injury with the more intense BP reduction arm in ATACH-2.
- Therefore, we recommend target SBP 140–160 mmHg.

2. Antihypertensive Regimens

Use titratable drugs such as nicardipine and labetalol.
- Nicardipine 5 mg/h and titrate up to 15 mg/h as needed.
- Labetalol 10–20 mg IV bolus, repeat as needed up to 60 mg. A labetalol infusion can also be started and titrated.
- Avoid nitroprusside, as it is a powerful vasodilator of both veins and arteries, which can lead to increased ICP.
- Other antihypertensive agents are usually not effective in the ED for accelerated hypertension associated with ICH.

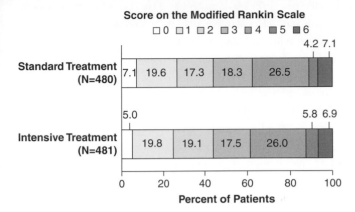

Figure 12.5 Distribution of modified Rankin scale (mRS) scores at 90 days in the two treatment groups of the ATACH-2 trial.
Source: ATACH-2 Trial Investigators, Neurological Emergency Treatment Trials Network. Intensive blood-pressure lowering in patients with acute cerebral hemorrhage. *N Engl J Med* 2016; 375: 1033–1043.[13] Copyright © 2016 Massachusetts Medical Society. Reproduced with permission from the Massachusetts Medical Society.

SURGICAL INTERVENTION

1. Surgical Clot Evacuation

Craniotomy with surgical evacuation of the hematoma helps prevent death from mass effect.

- There is no evidence that routine surgical clot evacuation results in improved outcome, as evidenced by the STICH and STICH-II trials.[14,15] It may be life-saving in the setting of impending herniation but does not result in improved functional outcome.
- Surgical clot evacuation is usually reserved for patients with the following:
  a. Younger age: no absolute cutoff but almost certainly < 75 years.

  b. Cerebellar hemorrhages of more than 3 cm causing displacement of
     the fourth ventricle; enlargement of the temporal horns (early
     obstructive hydrocephalus); compression of brainstem; decreased
     level of consciousness (but don't wait until the patient is comatose if
     the above criteria are met).
  c. Supratentorial hemorrhages with:
     ▪ Lobar or superficial location: close to brain surface.
     ▪ Volume > 20 mL with mass effect.
     ▪ Decreasing level of consciousness – drowsy but not comatose.
     ▪ More likely if not in eloquent location.

2. Ventriculostomy and CSF Drainage

Ventriculostomy and CSF drainage may be life-saving if obstructive
hydrocephalus is present.

3.   Decompressive Hemicraniectomy

In some cases, a decompressive hemicraniectomy without clot evacuation
is performed, offering a survival benefit to patients who have significant
mass effect and impending herniation.

4.   Minimally Invasive Techniques

Minimally invasive techniques include the stereotactic insertion of a catheter
and injection of tPA inside the clot to break it down. This is the basis of the
MISTIE trials.[16] MISTIE III demonstrated that catheter evacuation followed
by thrombolysis with tPA was safe but did not improve functional outcomes at
1 year. There was a suggestion of benefit in those in whom the residual clot
was reduced to 15 mL or less. Another technique, a parafascicular, trans-
sulcal approach (BrainPath) is currently being studied in the ENRICH trial.[17]
The hypothesis behind these minimally invasive techniques is that
minimizing the disruption of adjacent healthy fibers during clot evacuation
allows for better long-term functional outcomes.

OTHER ASPECTS OF ICH CARE

1. **Hydrocephalus management** – In cases of obstructive hydrocephalus from IVH or extrinsic mass effect of the hematoma onto the ventricular system, a ventriculostomy can be placed. This is more likely to be indicated if the third and fourth ventricles are filled with blood and if the exam is deteriorating. A ventriculostomy has the advantage of draining blood and CSF and provides a direct measure of ICP.
   - Goal ICP < 20 mmHg, goal CPP > 60 mmHg.
   - The goal is to reduce the ventriculomegaly and clear the third and fourth ventricles of blood.
   - In the CLEAR trials, instilling tPA in the ventricles to accelerate ventricular clot dissolution and drainage of CSF had a mortality benefit but was not associated with improved functional outcome in CLEAR III.[18]
   - A subgroup of patients with larger IVH volume (> 20 mL) were found to have significantly better functional outcome after intraventricular tPA therapy. This is basis for the design of the future CLEAR IV trial.

2. **Maintain euvolemia, normothermia**.

3. **Control ICP**
   - Head of bed > 30 degrees
   - Osmotherapy with mannitol or hypertonic solutions
   - Hyperventilation

4. **Watch for neurological deterioration** (see *Prognosis and Outcome*, below).

5. **Withhold full-dose anticoagulation for at least 2 weeks**.

6. **DVT prophylaxis**
   - Sequential compression devices to prevent DVT.[19]
   - Start SC heparin or LMWH for DVT prophylaxis 1–4 days after ictus, provided hematoma size stability has been established and coagulation parameters are normalized.[7]

7. **Seizure prophylaxis/treatment**
   - Early seizures (within the first week after bleed) occur in up to 31% of patients with ICH. More than half of those who seize do so in the first 24 hours.
   - Late seizures (beyond the first week) occur in up to 10% of patients and are related to the development of gliosis, leading to epilepsy.
   - Seizure prophylaxis in the early phase was not shown to alter functional outcome.[20] As a matter of fact, the use of phenytoin in this setting was associated with worse outcomes. This could be drug-specific however.
   - Lobar and cortical hemorrhages are more predisposed to seizures than deep hemorrhages.
   - Currently, guidelines do not support the routine prophylaxis of seizures after an ICH.[7]
   - Obviously, if a patient seizes, he/she needs to be treated. Duration of treatment will vary but is typically at least a couple of months.
8. **Talk with family** about expected quality of life, advance directives, withdrawal of support if appropriate.
9. **Start working on disposition early**: rehab consult, case manager.

■ Prognosis and Outcome

NEUROLOGICAL DETERIORATION IN ICH

(The ranking is our impression)

   Cause 1: rebleeding/hematoma expansion
   Cause 2: hydrocephalus (might itself be due to rebleeding)
   Cause 3: cerebral edema

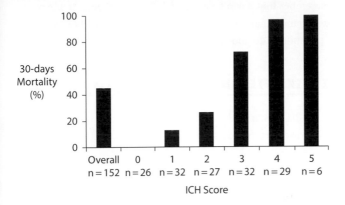

Figure 12.6 Increasing 30-day mortality with increasing ICH score.
Source: Hemphill JC, Bonovich DC, Besmertis L, *et al.* The ICH score: a simple, reliable grading scale for intracerebral hemorrhage. *Stroke* 2001; 32: 891–897.[22] Reproduced with permission.

Cause 4: general medical problems (infection, MI, electrolyte
imbalance, pulmonary emboli)

ICH OUTCOME

Correlates with initial GCS, size of hematoma, and presence of IVH.[21]
- GCS < 9 and ICH volume > 60 mL: 90% 1-month mortality
- GCS ≥ 9 and ICH volume < 30 mL: 17% 1-month mortality
- Also see the ICH score in Appendix 7 (Figure 12.6)[22]
    i.   ICH score ≥ 5: close to 100% 1-month mortality
    ii. ICH score ≥ 4: > 90% 1-month mortality
    iii. ICH score 2: 20–30% 1-month mortality
    iv. ICH score ≤ 1: < 15% 1-month mortality

But also remember that it can be a "self-fulfilling prophecy." If one treats with the expectation that the patient will do poorly (i.e., withdrawal of care), the patient will do poorly.

STROKE RISK AFTER INTRACEREBRAL HEMORRHAGE

Recurrence of ICH is estimated to be 1–2% per year.[23,24] It is not certain what the ischemic stroke occurrence risk in this population is, and it might be similar to ICH recurrence risk.[23,25,26] Instead of taking ICH as a group, consider the following factors relevant to ICH recurrence.

1. **Deep hemorrhages related to hypertension**:
   - Risk of ICH recurrence is lower.[23]
   - The PROGRESS trial showed that antihypertensive treatment significantly reduces risk of ICH.[27]
   - Therefore, in this population, once the blood pressure is in acceptable ranges, it may be reasonable to start antiplatelet therapy if the patient is at risk for ischemic vascular disease (coronary artery disease and ischemic stroke).

2. **Lobar hemorrhages**, which are often related to amyloid angiopathy in the elderly:
   - Further ICH recurrence risk can be estimated by using MRI MPGR/SWI sequence. The main utility of obtaining MRI of brain on elderly patients with ICH is to look for asymptomatic microhemorrhages on MPGR/SWI sequence.[28]
   - The greater the age and the number of microhemorrhages, the greater the certainty of amyloid angiopathy as the pathologic diagnosis.

3. **Hemorrhages related to vascular malformations**:
   - If not treated, they have a high recurrence risk, regardless of location (deep or lobar).

STARTING ANTIPLATELETS AND ANTICOAGULANTS AFTER INTRACEREBRAL HEMORRHAGE

When to resume (or initiate) antithrombotic therapy after an ICH is an area of intense debate in the scientific community. Most practitioners will wait for at least 2–4 weeks but this needs to be carefully weighed against the risk of thromboembolism. Conditions such as metallic prosthetic valves are high-risk for thromboembolism and therefore may require sooner anticoagulation.

- Left atrial appendage closure (e.g., Watchman device) is an alternative to anticoagulation in patients with atrial fibrillation who are at an unacceptable bleeding risk.
- If antiplatelet therapy is indicated to prevent subsequent ischemic events, there is no reason to start antiplatelet therapy in the first week or so after ICH. If the bleed had occurred on dual antiplatelet therapy (e.g., aspirin plus clopidogrel), the patient should be changed to monotherapy if possible.
- After warfarin-associated ICH, the decision to restart warfarin or a DOAC is based on the INR at the time of the bleed and the reason for warfarin. If INR was above or below the therapeutic range, a DOAC would be a logical alternative in patients with atrial fibrillation. If the patient has a prosthetic heart valve, the patient should return to anticoagulation as long as infectious endocarditis is ruled out.

References

1. LoPresti MA, Bruce SS, Camacho E, *et al*. Hematoma volume as the major determinant of outcomes after intracerebral hemorrhage. *J Neurol Sci* 2014; 345: 3–7.
2. Qureshi AI, Tuhrim S, Broderick JP, *et al*. Spontaneous intracerebral hemorrhage. *N Engl J Med* 2001; 344: 1450–1460.
3. Beslow LA, Ichord RN, Kasner SE, *et al*. ABC/XYZ estimates intracerebral hemorrhage volume as a percent of total brain volume in children. *Stroke* 2010; 41: 691–694.

4. Brott T, Broderick J, Kothari R, *et al.* Early hemorrhage growth in patients with intracerebral hemorrhage. *Stroke* 1997; 28: 1–5.

5. Al-Mufti F, Thabet AM, Singh T, *et al.* Clinical and radiographic predictors of intracerebral hemorrhage outcome. *Interv Neurol* 2018; 7: 118–136.

6. Morotti A, Brouwers HB, Romero JM, *et al.*; Antihypertensive Treatment of Acute Cerebral Hemorrhage II and Neurological Emergencies Treatment Trials Investigators. Intensive blood pressure reduction and spot sign in intracerebral hemorrhage: a secondary analysis of a randomized clinical trial. *JAMA Neurol* 2017; 74: 950–960. doi:10.1001/jamaneurol.2017.1014.

7. Hemphill JC, Greenberg SM, Anderson CS, *et al.* Guidelines for the management of spontaneous intracerebral hemorrhage: a guideline for healthcare professionals from the American Heart Association/American Stroke Association. *Stroke* 2015; 46: 2032–2060.

8. Mayer SA, Brun NC, Begtrup K, *et al.*; FAST Trial Investigators. Efficacy and safety of recombinant activated factor VII for acute intracerebral hemorrhage. *N Engl J Med* 2008; 358: 2127–2137.

9. Steiner T, Poli S, Griebe M, *et al.* Fresh frozen plasma versus prothrombin complex concentrate in patients with intracranial haemorrhage related to vitamin K antagonists (INCH): a randomised trial. *Lancet Neurol* 2016; 15: 566–573.

10. Baharoglu MI, Cordonnier C, Al-Shahi Salman R, *et al.*; PATCH Investigators. Platelet transfusion versus standard care after acute stroke due to spontaneous cerebral haemorrhage associated with antiplatelet therapy (PATCH): a randomised, open-label, phase 3 trial. *Lancet* 2016; 387: 2605–2613.

11. Butcher KS, Jeerakathil T, Hill M, *et al.*; ICH ADAPT Investigators. The Intracerebral Hemorrhage Acutely Decreasing Arterial Pressure trial. *Stroke* 2013; 44: 620–626.

12. Anderson CS, Heeley E, Huang Y, *et al.*; INTERACT2 Investigators. Rapid blood-pressure lowering in patients with acute intracerebral hemorrhage. *N Engl J Med* 2013; 368: 2355–2365.

13. Qureshi AI, Palesch YY, Barsan WG, *et al.*; ATACH-2 Trial Investigators, Neurological Emergency Treatment Trials Network. Intensive blood-pressure lowering in patients with acute cerebral hemorrhage. *N Engl J Med* 2016; 375: 1033–1043.

14. Mendelow AD, Gregson BA, Fernandes HM, *et al.*; STICH Investigators. Early surgery versus initial conservative treatment in patients with spontaneous supratentorial intracerebral haematomas in the International Surgical Trial in Intracerebral Haemorrhage (STICH): a randomised trial. *Lancet* 2005; 365: 387–397.

15. Mendelow AD, Gregson BA, Rowan EN, *et al.*; STICH II Investigators. Early surgery versus initial conservative treatment in patients with spontaneous supratentorial lobar intracerebral haematomas (STICH II): a randomised trial. *Lancet* 2013; 382: 397–408.

16. Hanley DF, Thompson RE, Rosenblum M, *et al.*; MISTIE III Investigators. Efficacy and safety of minimally invasive surgery with thrombolysis in intracerebral haemorrhage evacuation (MISTIE III): a randomised, controlled, open-label, blinded endpoint phase 3 trial. *Lancet* 2019; 393: 1021–1032. doi: 10.1016/S0140-6736(19)30195-3.

17. ENRICH: Early MiNimally-invasive Removal of IntraCerebral Hemorrhage (ICH) (ENRICH). *ClinicalTrials.gov*. https://clinicaltrials.gov/ct2/show/NCT02880878 (accessed June 2019).

18. Hanley DF, Lane K, McBee N, *et al.*; CLEAR III Investigators. Thrombolytic removal ofintraventricular haemorrhage in treatment of severe stroke: results of the randomised, multicentre, multiregion, placebo-controlled CLEAR III trial. *Lancet* 2017; 389: 603–611.

19. Lacut K, Bressollette L, Le Gal G, *et al.*; VICTORIAh Investigators. Prevention of venous thrombosis in patients with acute intracerebral hemorrhage. *Neurology* 2005; 65: 865–869.

20. Messé SR, Sansing LH, Cucchiara BL, *et al.*; CHANT Investigators. Prophylactic antiepileptic drug use is associated with poor outcome following ICH. *Neurocrit Care* 2009; 11: 38–44.

21. Broderick JP, Brott TG, Duldner JE, Tomsick T, Huster G. Volume of intracerebral hemorrhage: a powerful and easy-to-use predictor of 30-day mortality. *Stroke* 1993; 24: 987–993.

22. Hemphill JC, Bonovich DC, Besmertis L, Manley GT, Johnston SC. The ICH score: a simple, reliable grading scale for intracerebral hemorrhage. *Stroke* 2001; 32: 891–897.

23. Bailey RD, Hart RG, Benavente O, Pearce LA. Recurrent brain hemorrhage is more frequent than ischemic stroke after intracranial hemorrhage. *Neurology* 2001; 56: 773–777.

24. Hanger HC, Wilkinson TJ, Fayez-Iskander N, Sainsbury R. The risk of recurrent stroke after intracerebral haemorrhage. *J Neurol Neurosurg Psychiatry* 2007; 78: 836–840.

25. Azarpazhooh MR, Nicol MB, Donnan GA, *et al.* Patterns of stroke recurrence according to subtype of first stroke event: the North East Melbourne Stroke Incidence Study (NEMESIS). *Int J Stroke* 2008; 3: 158–164.

26. Zia E, Engström G, Svensson PJ, Norrving B, Pessah-Rasmussen H. Three-year survival and stroke recurrence rates in patients with primary intracerebral hemorrhage. *Stroke* 2009; 40: 3567–3573.

27. PROGRESS Collaborative Group. Randomised trial of a perindopril-based blood-pressure-lowering regimen among 6,105 individuals with previous stroke or transient ischaemic attack. *Lancet* 2001; 358: 1033–1041.

28. Greenberg SM, Eng JA, Ning M, Smith EE, Rosand J. Hemorrhage burden predicts recurrent intracerebral hemorrhage after lobar hemorrhage. *Stroke* 2004; 35: 1415–1420.

13

Subarachnoid Hemorrhage

This chapter covers the diagnosis and management of spontaneous subarachnoid hemorrhage due to rupture of intracranial aneurysms. At the end of the chapter we also discuss unruptured intracranial aneurysms. Much SAH management is not based on good-quality evidence. Much of what is recommended here comes from published practice guidelines and what is commonly practiced.[1] Options for therapy might be limited by the availability and experience of persons performing surgery, endovascular therapy, and neurointensive care.

■ Definition

Subarachnoid hemorrhage (SAH) is bleeding into the subarachnoid space around the brain. Trauma is the most common cause of SAH. We do not discuss traumatic SAH in this chapter. This chapter covers spontaneous SAH, 80% of which are due to intracranial saccular aneurysms.

■ Epidemiology

- 3% of all strokes but 5% of stroke deaths.
- Incidence 10–15 per 100 000 person-years in the USA, with higher risk among African-Americans. Worldwide, higher incidence reported in Japan and Scandinavia.[2]

- Females have higher incidence (60% of patients are female).
- Modifiable risk factors: hypertension, tobacco use, oral contraceptives, alcohol, and stimulants.
- Non-modifiable risk factors: older age (peak is 50–60 years old), female sex.
- Other diseases associated with aneurysms: polycystic kidney disease, Marfan syndrome, Ehlers–Danlos syndrome, coarctation of the aorta, fibromuscular dysplasia.
- Location: 30% anterior communicating, 25% posterior communicating, 20% MCAs, 10% basilar, 5% vertebral, and 25% have multiple aneurysms.

■ Presentation

- "The worst headache of my life."
- Thunderclap headache.
- Headache is sometimes associated with focal neurological symptoms such as CN III palsy or appendicular motor deficits.
- Neck stiffness.
- Photophobia.
- Various degrees of unresponsiveness, from awake to comatose.

■ Diagnosis

As this condition is potentially life-threatening, diagnostic evaluation should be done emergently.

DIAGNOSIS OF SUBARACHNOID HEMORRHAGE

- **CT of the head without contrast**
  - In the first 6 hours, the sensitivity of non-contrast CT is 100%. By 72 hours, it is > 97% and, by day 5, it goes down to about 50%.

- If head CT is normal, but you have a high clinical suspicion for SAH, you must do a lumbar puncture, because CT can miss small or subtle SAHs, especially if more than 72 hours has passed since the ictus.[3]
- **Lumbar puncture**
  - Don't forget to personally examine the fluid for xanthochromia. Compare the color to water. Measure red blood cells in first and last tube collected. Also, it is often helpful to personally deliver the tubes of CSF to the lab to make sure that they are processed quickly.
  - The other parameters in the CSF (glucose, protein, WBC) will help you rule out meningitis.
- **MRI brain**
  - GRE or SWI sequence on MRI can detect old SAH.
  - FLAIR sequence shows acute SAH very well.

DIAGNOSIS OF INTRACRANIAL ANEURYSMS

- **Digital subtraction angiography (DSA)** – the gold standard. If the DSA is negative and the suspicion for aneurysm is high, repeating the DSA in a few days can increase the yield by 10%.
- **CT angiography (CTA)** – sensitivity 98%, but depends on CT equipment. Difficult to see aneurysms near bones.
- **MR angiography (MRA)** – fair test for screening for unruptured aneurysms > 5 mm.

CAUSES OF SAH OTHER THAN INTRACRANIAL ANEURYSMS

- **Perimesencephalic SAH** – blood limited to anterior to midbrain (or pons) and can reach the medial aspects of the sylvian fissures. Angiogram is negative for aneurysms. The cause of the bleed is unknown (venous?). It carries a good prognosis and a benign course.

- **Arteriovenous malformation (AVM)** – it classically causes intraparenchymal hemorrhage, but it can lead to SAH. DSA will help in diagnosis.
- **Arterial dissection (vertebral artery usually)** – arterial dissection that extends from the extracranial to the intracranial portion of an artery or is limited to the intracranial artery can lead to SAH. This can occur spontaneously or it may be post-traumatic. DSA and MRI can be helpful in visualizing the abnormality.
- **Arteriovenous fistula** – can be seen only with careful DSA.
- **Pituitary apoplexy** – MRI is helpful in making the diagnosis.
- **Sympathetic mimetic agents (e.g., cocaine)** – can lead to SAH, ICH, or cerebral ischemia.
- **Trauma** – detailed history or external head examination may suggest trauma as the primary cause. Often located along convexities or in association with subdural hematoma.
- **Vasculitis** – difficult to diagnose, since DSA is neither sensitive nor specific and brain biopsy is specific but insensitive.

■ Management of Ruptured Aneurysms

GOALS

- Prevention of rebleeding.
- Treatment of the aneurysm itself: clipping or coiling.
- Prevention and treatment of complications: hydrocephalus, seizure, cardiac ischemia or arrhythmia, vasospasm, hyponatremia, infections, DVTs.
- Rehabilitation.

PREVENTION OF REBLEEDING

- Rebleeding is maximal in the first 24 hours after SAH (4%). It carries a high mortality.

- Securing the aneurysm with coiling or clipping as early as possible is the single most important preventive measure against rebleeding.
- Independent predictors of rebleeding are: pre-existing hypertension, basilar artery location of the aneurysm, size ≥ 9 mm, acute hydrocephalus, and presence of ICH.[4]
- The following measures are often taken, but without much evidence:
  - Blood-pressure control is important before definitive treatment to reduce rebleeding. MAP goal is 70–100 mmHg, significantly lower than with other stroke syndromes.
  - Bed rest in ICU with monitoring.
  - Prevention of pain, nausea/vomiting, straining/constipation, dyssynchrony with the ventilator.
- Antifibrinolytic drugs (epsilon-aminocaproic acid, tranexamic acid) reduce rebleeding but promote ischemic/thromboembolic complications, and therefore their use is usually limited to 72 hours or until the aneurysm gets treated. These drugs are rarely used, because of their complications.

TREATMENT OF THE ANEURYSM ITSELF

This should be done as early as possible, especially in patients with mild to moderate clinical deficits, since the goal is to prevent rebleeding.

1. Surgical Clipping

Craniotomy and placement of a metal clip takes the aneurysm out of the arterial circulation.

- It is believed to be the best way to prevent aneurysmal bleeding long-term.
- **More advantageous than coiling if:**
  a. the aneurysm has a wide neck (high neck-to-dome ratio).
  b. the aneurysm is either large (> 15 mm) or giant (> 24 mm).

    c. the SAH is associated with an intraparenchymal clot that needs evacuation.

    d. the aneurysm is located too distally and is therefore not accessible by endovascular means.

    e. multiple aneurysms need treatment.

- **Drawbacks of the procedure**:

    a. Aneurysms in the posterior circulation are not easily amenable to open surgery.

    b. Requires general anesthesia, and therefore patients with comorbidities may not be good candidates.

    c. Carries higher mortality/morbidity rate than coiling.

2. Endovascular Coiling

Coiling has become the alternative treatment. When you fill the aneurysm with coils, it thromboses, and effectively takes the aneurysm out of the arterial circulation.

- **Advantages**:

    a. Subsequent rebleed rate is not as low as with surgical clipping, but pretty close.

    b. Can address posterior circulation aneurysms.

    c. Less invasive and carries less mortality/morbidity than clipping.

- **Disadvantages**:

    a. Not as durable as clipping. Long-term data are not available.

    b. Complete obliteration of the aneurysm is not always achieved initially and may require repeat intervention. Higher rate of rebleeding than clipping.

    c. Some aneurysms are not amenable to coiling due to distal location or shape (wide neck). Having said that, new technologies such as stent-assisted coiling and flow-diversion devices have allowed treatment of wide-necked and complex or large/giant aneurysms endovascularly.

3. Clipping or Coiling?

That is the big question. Cases should be individualized based on clinical features, anatomy, and expertise of local surgical and endovascular personnel.

- ISAT was a randomized multicenter trial comparing the two methods:[5]
  a. 23.7% of coiled versus 30.6% of clipped patients were dependent or dead at 1 year (absolute risk reduction of a bad outcome: 6.9%).
  b. For this trial, the patients were required to be good candidates for both procedures (~60% were treated outside the trial). 88% of patients had mild SAH (WFNS grade 1 or 2 – see Appendix 7). Therefore, the results may not be generalizable to the entire population of SAH patients.
  c. Locations: 51% were ACA or anterior communicating artery (AcomA) and 33% were ICA or posterior communicating artery (PcomA) aneurysms. Only 14% were MCA aneurysms and 2.7% were posterior circulation aneurysms.
  d. Presumably, most MCA aneurysms were clipped and posterior circulation aneurysms coiled outside of the study.

Based on ISAT, the preferred treatment of many ruptured ACA, ICA, AcomA, or PcomA aneurysms is coiling, but, as already stated, the approach must be individualized based on many factors that are beyond the scope of this text (Figure 13.1). Expert multidisciplinary consultation is needed, which underscores the need for these patients to be managed at specialized referral centers.

PREVENTION AND TREATMENT OF COMPLICATIONS

As with other strokes, general medical complications such as DVT, pneumonia, and other infections are common. SAH also has its own particular complications: hydrocephalus, seizure, cerebral vasospasm, and delayed ischemic deficits.

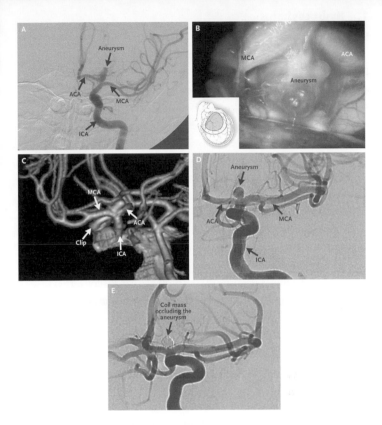

Figure 13.1 Terminal ICA aneurysm before and after treatment. Panels A, B, C are from a patient who underwent clipping (respectively: DSA pre-treatment; at the time of clipping; post-clipping CTA with reconstruction). Panels D and E refer to another patient who underwent coiling (respectively: before and after treatment). (A black and white version of this figure will appear in some formats. For the color version, please refer to the plate section.)

Source: Lawton MT, Vates GE. Subarachnoid hemorrhage. *N Engl J Med* 2017; 377: 257–266.[6] Copyright ©2017 Massachusetts Medical Society. Reproduced with permission from the Massachusetts Medical Society.

1. Hydrocephalus

Significant hydrocephalus occurs in ~20% of patients with SAH. This may be already present at the time of presentation with SAH. Hydrocephalus and vasospasm are more often than not found in association, possibly because of their relation to the amount of subarachnoid blood.

- **Diagnosis**
  - Clinical signs include a decrease in level of consciousness, agitation, hypertension, and bradycardia. However, these signs are not specific.
  - CT of head without contrast: enlargement of ventricles.
- **Treatment**
  - External drainage of CSF via intraventricular catheter (ventriculostomy or external ventricular drain).
  - Ventriculostomy must be monitored for amount of CSF drained and for infection.
  - If hydrocephalus is persistent, CSF drainage can be converted to internal drainage by placement of ventriculoperitoneal, ventriculoatrial, or lumboperitoneal shunt by a neurosurgeon.

2. Seizures

Seizures may increase blood pressure and may increase rebleeding risk.

- **Prevention**
  - Without good evidence for efficacy, we do not routinely administer antiepileptic agents unless a seizure has occurred – or, if we do, it is only for a short time (3–5 days).
  - Regimens: phenytoin 300 mg per day and adjusted to maintain level of 10–20 µg/mL. Or levetiracetam 500–1000 mg bid.
- **Diagnosis**
  - Non-convulsive seizure may go unrecognized. Bedside EEG may help if SAH itself or sedative drugs affect assessment.

- **Treatment**
  - Phenytoin is most commonly used and is available in intravenous and oral formulations. Among other anticonvulsants, levetiracetam, valproic acid, lacosamide, and phenobarbital are available in IV formulation.

3. Cerebral Vasospasm and Delayed Cerebral Ischemia (DCI)

Onset usually 3–5 days after SAH, maximal at 5–10 days, and can go on for 14 days. The typical window for vasospasm is therefore 4–14 days, but some patients experience an earlier onset, and vasospasm can extend past 2 weeks for others. Approximately 30% of SAH patients develop vasospasm, and 15–20% go on to have ischemic strokes. Predictors of DCI include poor admission neurological grade and severity of subarachnoid hemorrhage on initial non-contrast CT.

- **Prevention** – Vasospasm is unlikely to be the sole cause of DCI, since it can happen in patients who do not have angiographic evidence of vasospasm. Possible pathogenic mechanisms under investigation include: neuroinflammation, microcirculation dysregulation, microthrombosis, and cortical spreading depolarizations.
  a. **Calcium channel blockers** – nimodipine (Nimotop) 60 mg PO every 4 hours for 21 days. Adjust dose downwards and more frequent to 30 mg PO every 2 hours if blood pressure falls so low that adequate CPP is endangered. This should be started early after diagnosis of SAH to prevent vasospasm. It is important to realize that nimodipine was shown to improve functional outcome at 90 days but does not significantly reverse angiographic vasospasm.[7]
  b. **Maintenance of euvolemia** – We recommend Foley placement, especially in patients who are in vasospasm, with strict intake and output monitoring. In patients with hemodynamic compromise, more invasive hemodynamic monitoring may be required to maintain adequate fluid balance.[8]

    c. **Prevention of hypotension**

    d. **Magnesium sulfate** was not shown to improve functional outcome in the IMASH trial.[9]

    e. **Statins** were not found to reduce cerebral vasospasm, incidence of DCI, or poor outcome.[10]

- **Diagnosis**

    a. **TCD** (Appendix 2) – Velocity trend with daily or sequential measurements is more useful than one-time snapshot of velocities. So get a baseline and follow daily. Increasing flow velocity (> 120 cm/s) may indicate either vasospasm or hyperemia. In order to differentiate between the two, we calculate the Lindegaard ratio, which is the velocity ratio of MCA to extracranial ICA. An elevated Lindegaard ratio (> 3) indicates MCA vasospasm.

    b. **CTA** – Requires iodine contrast injection but may be combined with CT perfusion to diagnose vasospasm and ischemia.

    c. **Angiography (DSA)** – More invasive, but can also be linked to treatment with angioplasty or intra-arterial papaverine, nicardipine, or verapamil.

    d. **Clinical symptoms and signs** – Focal deficits similar to ischemic stroke. In addition, may have bilateral frontal lobe dysfunction (more cognitive and personality changes) in the case of anterior communicating artery vasospasm, or decreased level of consciousness if vertebrobasilar. You want to diagnose and treat vasospasm before these symptoms and signs develop.

- **Treatment**

    a. Hypertension – hypervolemia – hemodilution (triple-H therapy) used to be the dogma. Nowadays, we understand that blood-pressure augmentation is likely the most important element in this triad, and the other two have fallen out of favor. Fluid resuscitation in combination with pressors may be needed to bring the MAP up to 100–120 mmHg or more in order to reverse the vasospasm and prevent the development of an ischemic stroke.[11]

b. If vasospasm does not respond to blood-pressure augmentation, direct endovascular treatment can be performed with balloon angioplasty or infusion of a calcium channel blocker.

PROGNOSIS

- Refer to Appendix 7 for the Hunt and Hess scale and the World Federation of Neurologic Surgeons (WFNS) grading system.
- **Mortality** – 10–15% of patients with ruptured aneurysms die before reaching medical attention.[12] A quarter of the deaths are directly attributable to initial bleed, another quarter to vasospasm, and another quarter to rebleeding. In one study of 1200 hospitalized SAH patients, 18% died during the hospitalization, of whom 50% were do-not-resuscitate and had life support withdrawn at the time of cardiac death, and 42% were diagnosed with brain death.[13]
- **Morbidity** – one-third of patients have neurological deficit (Table 13.1).[14]
- **Rebleeding risk** – with unclipped aneurysms, 6% rebleed within the first 3 days, and 12% in the first 2 weeks.[15] Hypertension increases the chance of rebleeding.

ADMISSION SEQUENCE

The usual sequence of events upon admitting a patient who has suffered an SAH is as follows:

1. Establish diagnosis of SAH with CT or lumbar puncture as soon as possible.
2. Blood-pressure control, prophylactic anticonvulsants.
3. Neurosurgery consult, admission to ICU.

Table 13.1 One-month outcome after SAH by clinical status at presentation

Clinical status at presentation		Poor outcome (severe neurological deficits, vegetative, or dead)	Relative risk of poor outcome (95% CI)
Hunt & Hess scale	Grade I	22%	1
	Grade II	22%	1.0 (0.4–2.2)
	Grade III	50%	2.2 (1.1–10.9)
	Grade IV	87%	3.9 (2.3–7.8)
	Grade V	100%	∞
Glasgow Coma Scale	13–15	24%	1
	9–12	84%	3.6 (2.4–5.2)
	3–8	97%	4.1 (2.9–5.8)

Adapted from: Longstreth WT, Nelson LM, Koepsell TD, van Belle G. Clinical course of spontaneous subarachnoid hemorrhage: a population-based study in King County, Washington. *Neurology* 1993; 43: 712–718.[14]

- If necessary, transfer emergently to an appropriate hospital that has adequate neurosurgical, neurointerventional (coiling), and neurocritical care capability.
- Consider ventriculostomy if hydrocephalus is present.

4. Determine location of ruptured aneurysm with CTA or DSA (do on the first day).
5. Definitive aneurysm treatment (coiling or clipping).
6. Enteral nimodipine.
7. Watch for and treat vasospasm (first 2 weeks).
8. Anticipate non-neurological complications such as hemodynamic complications (Takotsubo cardiomyopathy, neurogenic pulmonary edema, arrhythmias) and hyponatremia (from SIADH or cerebral salt wasting) and treat them accordingly.

■ Unruptured Aneurysms

Unruptured aneurysms are sometimes found incidentally as part of brain imaging or because of neurological symptoms other than rupture and SAH. Some patients with SAH are found to have other aneurysms that have not ruptured. Some unruptured aneurysms are found through screening of those with a family history of SAH.

DIAGNOSIS

The diagnostic strategy is the same as for ruptured aneurysms, with DSA being the gold standard for accurate diagnosis and measurement of an aneurysm. CTA and MRA are fair screening tools.

NATURAL HISTORY

- 0.5–1% of the general population harbor unruptured intracranial aneurysms.
- Aneurysms often enlarge over time, especially in cases of uncontrolled hypertension and ongoing tobacco use.
- Controversy exists among experts about the natural course, and about whether and when to intervene.[16,17]
- **ISUIA study**
   a. The rupture rates were higher for aneurysms of larger size, in the posterior circulation (posterior communicating, posterior cerebral, vertebral, or basilar artery), and in patients with a history of previous SAH.[17]
   b. Among those with no history of SAH:
      ▪ Bleed rate ~0.1% per year if < 7 mm diameter

- Bleed rate ~0.5% per year if 7–12 mm diameter in anterior circulation
- Bleed rate ~3% per year if 7–12 mm diameter in posterior circulation
- Bleed rate > 3% per year if > 12 mm diameter

- **Other observational studies**
  a. Bleed rate 1–2% per year.
  b. The controversy and uncertainty of management depends on the paradoxical observation that despite the low rates of rupture of small aneurysms when followed over time, most subarachnoid hemorrhages are due to small aneurysms.

MANAGEMENT

The decision to clip or coil an unruptured aneurysm depends on five main factors:

1. **Previous history of bleeding** – increases risk of recurrence and weighs in favor of intervention, either clipping or coiling.
2. **Aneurysm location** – anterior circulation has less rupture risk and has less surgical morbidity.
3. **Aneurysm size** – unruptured aneurysms > 7 mm are more likely to bleed.
4. **Patient age** – increased morbidity with any intervention with increased age. Morbidity risk associated with coiling appears to be less dependent on age.
5. **Surgical experience** – perioperative and peri-coiling morbidity is lower in experienced hands.

Treatment decisions for each patient must be individualized by neurology, neurosurgery, and endovascular consultants based on these five variables. We are awaiting definitive data from ongoing trials that will provide more information to assist in our decisions, but the following are "general" recommendations:

1. Unruptured aneurysm cavernous or < 5–7 mm: leave alone.
2. Unruptured aneurysm > 5–7 mm, anterior circulation, patient < 65 years old, experienced surgeon/center: surgical clipping.
3. Unruptured aneurysm > 5–7 mm, posterior circulation, patient > 65 years old, experienced endovascular team: coiling.

References

1. Connolly ES, Rabinstein AA, Carhuapoma JR, *et al.* Guidelines for the management of aneurysmal subarachnoid hemorrhage: a guideline for healthcare professionals from the American Heart Association/American Stroke Association. *Stroke* 2012; 43: 1711–1737.
2. Labovitz DL, Halim AX, Brent B, *et al.* Subarachnoid hemorrhage incidence among Whites, Blacks and Caribbean Hispanics: the Northern Manhattan Study. *Neuroepidemiology* 2006; 26: 147–150.
3. Suarez JI, Tarr RW, Selman WR. Aneurysmal subarachnoid hemorrhage. *N Engl J Med* 2006; 354: 387–396.
4. Darkwah Oppong M, Gümüs M, Piersclanek D, *et al.* Aneurysm rebleeding before therapy: a predictable disaster? *J Neurosurg* 2018. doi:10.3171/2018.7.JNS181119. [Epub ahead of print]
5. Molyneux A, Kerr R, Stratton I, *et al.* International Subarachnoid Aneurysm Trial (ISAT) of neurosurgical clipping versus endovascular coiling in 2143 patients with ruptured intracranial aneurysms: a randomised trial. *Lancet* 2002; 360: 1267–1274.
6. Lawton MT, Vates GE. Subarachnoid hemorrhage. *N Engl J Med* 2017; 377: 257–266.
7. Petruk KC, West M, Mohr G, *et al.* Nimodipine treatment in poor-grade aneurysm patients: results of a multicenter double-blind placebo-controlled trial. *J Neurosurg* 1988; 68: 505–517.
8. van der Jagt M. Fluid management of the neurological patient: a concise review. *Crit Care* 2016; 20: 126.
9. van den Bergh WM, Algra A, van Kooten F, *et al.* Magnesium sulfate in aneurysmal subarachnoid hemorrhage: a randomized controlled trial. *Stroke* 2005; 36: 1011–1015.
10. Kirkpatrick PJ, Turner CL, Smith C, Hutchinson PJ, Murray GD;STASH Collaborators. Simvastatin in aneurysmal subarachnoid haemorrhage (STASH): a multicentre randomised phase 3 trial. *Lancet Neurol* 2014; 13: 666–675.

11. Muench E, Horn P, Bauhuf C, *et al.* Effects of hypervolemia and hypertension on regional cerebral blood flow, intracranial pressure, and brain tissue oxygenation after subarachnoid hemorrhage. *Crit Care Med* 2007; 35: 1844–1851.

12. Truelsen T, Bonita R, Duncan J, Anderson NE, Mee E. Changes in subarachnoid hemorrhage mortality, incidence, and case fatality in New Zealand between 1981–1983 and 1991–1993. *Stroke* 1998; 29: 2298–2303.

13. Lantigua H, Ortega-Gutierrez S, Schmidt JM, *et al.* Subarachnoid hemorrhage: who dies, and why? *Crit Care* 2015; 19: 309.

14. Longstreth WT, Nelson LM, Koepsell TD, van Belle G. Clinical course of spontaneous subarachnoid hemorrhage: a population-based study in King County, Washington. *Neurology* 1993; 43: 712–718.

15. Kassell NF, Torner JC, Jane JA, Haley EC, Adams HP. The International Cooperative Study on the Timing of Aneurysm Surgery. Part 2: surgical results. *J Neurosurg* 1990; 73: 37–47.

16. International Study of Unruptured Intracranial Aneurysms Investigators. Unruptured intracranial aneurysms: risk of rupture and risks of surgical intervention. *N Engl J Med* 1998; 339: 1725–1733.

17. Wiebers DO, Whisnant JP, Huston J, *et al.*; International Study of Unruptured Intracranial Aneurysms Investigators. Unruptured intracranial aneurysms: natural history, clinical outcome, and risks of surgical and endovascular treatment. *Lancet* 2003; 362: 103–110.

14

Organization of Stroke Care

As acute stroke therapies have developed, the context in which stroke care is provided has become more important. Creating and maintaining the organization of stroke care within a region or even a hospital requires much commitment and effort. High-quality stroke care requires coordination and communication between multiple stakeholders in the prehospital and in-hospital settings in what the American Heart Association (AHA) and American Stroke Association (ASA) term the "stroke chain of survival" (Table 14.1).[1] An ASA task force offers a set of recommendations on systems of stroke care.[2,3] The European Stroke Initiative also provides a good set of evidence-based recommendations.[4-6]

■ Timely Care

Time is a crucial factor in improving stroke outcomes. Most investigational therapies for hemorrhagic stroke are also focused on early interventions. Treatments for acute ischemic stroke (AIS) are time-sensitive. Intravenous tPA must be given within 4.5 hours. Endovascular thrombolysis (EVT) must be initiated within 6 hours for most patients, with imaging-selected patients eligible up to 24 hours. Both IV tPA and EVT for AIS are most effective when initiated early, and ideally within the first hour of symptoms onset.[7,8] However, only 3–9% of AIS patients receive IV

Table 14.1 Stroke chain of survival

Detection	Patient or bystander recognition of stroke signs and symptoms
Dispatch	Immediate activation of 9-1-1 and priority EMS dispatch
Delivery	Prompt triage and transport to most appropriate stroke hospital and prehospital notification
Door	Immediate ED triage to high-acuity area
Data	Prompt ED evaluation, stroke team activation, laboratory studies, and brain imaging
Decision	Diagnosis and determination of most appropriate therapy; discussion with patient and family
Drug	Administration of appropriate drugs or other interventions
Disposition	Timely admission to stroke unit, intensive care unit, or transfer

ED, emergency department; EMS, emergency medical services.

Source: Jauch EC, Saver JL, Adams HP, *et al.* Guidelines for the early management of patients with acute ischemic stroke. *Stroke* 2013; 44: 870–947 (Table 3, page 873).[1] Reproduced with permission.

thrombolysis and far fewer EVT, which is due to a combination of delays in recognition of stroke symptoms, activation of EMS, prehospital triage, and in-hospital stroke expertise.[9-11] Therefore a focus on expediting prehospital stroke care is key.

■ Prehospital Stroke Care

- **Promotion of public awareness** – Patients, families, and the general public must be educated regarding stroke symptom recognition, available stroke therapies, and the importance of emergency medical care. Several studies have demonstrated an increase in stroke symptom knowledge and readiness to call 911 through dynamic educational interventions with both children and adults.[12-14]

- **Mobile stroke units** – The concept of a mobile stroke unit (MSU) to expedite prehospital evaluation and treatment of acute stroke patients was first developed in the early 2000s in Homberg/Saarland, Germany.[15] An MSU is a specialized stroke ambulance equipped with a CT scanner for on-board brain imaging, laboratory testing, either an on-board or remote (via telemedicine) vascular neurologist, tPA, and commonly administered medications. There are more than 20 MSUs now worldwide, with an ongoing comparative effectiveness trial led by investigators in Houston, Texas, evaluating prehospital IV tPA treatment with MSU compared to standard in-hospital care.[16]

- **Partnership with prehospital providers** – Dispatch personnel, ambulance drivers, emergency medical technicians, paramedics, and their medical supervisors must agree to prioritize acute stroke and train to increase stroke recognition. Acute stroke patients must be evaluated in a timely fashion, and preferentially transported to a stroke center if one is available. Ideally, prehospital providers prenotify the receiving facility or stroke team directly and shorten the time to evaluation. ED physicians should evaluate immediately upon patient arrival. Stroke team members should be notified at the earliest time possible.

■ Prehospital Stroke Scales

In order for patients to receive the appropriate treatment quickly they must be transported to a hospital that can provide acute stroke care including IV thrombolysis and in the case of large-vessel occlusion (LVO) also EVT.

Several prehospital stroke scales have been utilized by medics in the field to help identify patients who are more likely to have had a stroke. The most studied of these scales are the Cincinnati Prehospital Stroke Severity Scale (CPSSS), the Los Angeles Motor Scale (LAMS), and the Rapid Arterial

Occlusion Evaluation (RACE) (Table 14.2). In a prehospital scale that aims to predict LVO, cortical signs (speech difficulty, gaze deviation, and neglect) may be more sensitive than motor deficits.[17]

■ Drip-and-Ship versus Mothership Models

Currently, in most major cities, the "drip-and-ship" model of care is utilized, in which eligible AIS patients are transported to the nearest hospital, treated with IV tPA, and then transferred to a high-volume tertiary center for EVT evaluation and ongoing acute stroke care.[25] In the "mothership" model of care, patients with suspected LVOs are transported directly from the field by EMS to EVT-capable centers.[26] Observational registry data suggest that the drip-and-ship model may be associated with delayed treatment and worse outcomes in patients who require interhospital transfer. The ongoing prospective randomized RACECAT in Barcelona, Spain, is comparing the drip-and-ship versus mothership models of care for AIS patients with suspected LVO.[27]

■ Stroke Centers

Whenever possible, stroke patients should be treated in hospitals with the ability to deliver acute stroke treatments quickly and efficiently. It is important to foster the development of such "stroke centers." This may involve the need to establish a regional organization of stroke care.

Primary stroke centers (PSCs) are hospitals that have sufficient medical providers, protocols, and facilities to provide good basic acute stroke care, with acute stroke teams, stroke units, and ability to administer IV TPA. In the USA the Brain Attack Coalition has published criteria for PSCs,[28] and the Joint Commission on Accreditation of Healthcare Organizations started accreditation of primary stroke centers in December 2003.[29]

Table 14.2 Overview of LVO prediction scales

	No. of patients	No. of items	Items	Cutoff	Need to calculate score	SENS	SPEC	ACC
3-ISS	171	3	Level of consciousness Gaze deviation Motor function	≥ 4	Yes	0.67	0.92	0.86
CPSSS	303	3	Level of consciousness Gaze deviation Arm weakness	≥ 2	Yes	0.83	0.40	0.67
FAST-ED	727	6	Facial palsy Arm weakness Speech changes Eye deviation Denial/neglect	≥ 4	Yes	0.60	0.89	0.79
LAMS	94	3	Facial palsy Arm drift Grip strength	≥ 4	Yes	0.69	0.81	0.77
RACE	357	6	Facial palsy Arm motor function Leg motor function Head and gaze deviation Aphasia Agnosia	≥ 5	Yes	0.85	0.68	0.82

Table 14.2 (cont.)

	No. of patients	No. of items	Items	Cutoff	Need to calculate score	SENS	SPEC	ACC
PASS	3127	3	Level of consciousness Gaze palsy/deviation Arm weakness	≥ 2	Yes	0.66	0.83	0.74
VAN	62	4	Arm weakness Visual disturbance Aphasia Neglect	No	No	1.0	0.90	0.92

Adapted from: Beume LA, Hieber, M, Kaller CP, *et al.* Large vessel occlusion in acute stroke: cortical symptoms are more sensitive prehospital indicators than motor deficits. *Stroke* 2018; 49: 2323–2329. doi: 10.1161/STROKEAHA.118.022253.[17]

3-ISS, 3-Item Stroke Scale;[18] CPSSS, Cincinnati Prehospital Stroke Severity Scale;[19] FAST-ED, Field Assessment Stroke Triage for Emergency Destination;[20] LAMS, Los Angeles Motor Scale;[21] RACE, Rapid Arterial oCclusion Evaluation;[22] PASS, Prehospital Acute Severity Scale;[23] VAN, Stroke Vision, Aphasia, Neglect assessment;[24] SENS, sensitivity; SPEC, specificity; ACC, accuracy.

Comprehensive stroke centers have advanced capability with availability of interventionalists and neurosurgeons. Quality-assurance measures such as written protocols and performance measurements should be part of stroke centers.

■ Telemedicine for Stroke (Telestroke)

In hospitals where physicians with expertise in stroke are not available, especially in rural areas where they are often many miles away, consultation by telephone or preferably real-time video conference system (telemedicine) allows safe administration of thrombolytics locally. It also can help identify appropriate patients requiring transfer to a comprehensive stroke center. Telemedicine is more accurate (> 95% accuracy) in diagnosing stroke and tPA eligibility than telephone (75%).[30] Implementation of hyperacute telemedicine for stroke (telestroke) consultations by a vascular neurologist increases the use of IV tPA at community hospitals, with no difference in complication rates as compared to in person consultation.[31,32]

■ Stroke Teams

Acute stroke teams help provide the above care based on the latest evidence-based guidelines. The team might consist of neurologists, internists, ED physicians, neurosurgeons, intensivists, rehabilitation physicians, endovascular neurointerventionists, ultrasonographers, nurses, therapists, dieticians, patient care managers, smoking cessation counselors, stroke educators, etc. Stroke care should be optimized to meet the needs of the local region and institution.

■ Stroke Units

Specialized stroke units have been shown to improve outcomes. Patients cared for on stroke units are more likely to be alive and living independently 1 year after stroke.[33] Therefore, all acute stroke patients should ideally be admitted to a stroke unit. Some uncertainty exists regarding what features of the stroke unit are important; however, care on a discrete ward is associated with improved outcomes. Comprehensive stroke units should have trained nurses, therapists (physical, occupational, speech), and physicians acting in a multidisciplinary approach. Acute stroke care units in the North American model can take care of tPA-treated patients. This includes frequent monitoring of vital signs, cardiac rhythm monitoring, and the ability to administer some intravenous antihypertensive drugs.

References

1. Jauch EC, Saver JL, Adams HP, *et al*. Guidelines for the early management of patients with acute ischemic stroke: a guideline for healthcare professionals from the American Heart Association/American Stroke Association. *Stroke* 2013; 44: 870–947. doi:10.1161/STR.0b013e318284056a.

2. Schwamm LH, Pancioli A, Acker JE, *et al*. Recommendations for the establishment of stroke systems of care: recommendations from the American Stroke Association's Task Force on the Development of Stroke Systems. *Stroke* 2005; 36: 690–703.

3. Higashida R, Alberts MJ, Alexander DN, *et al*. Interactions within stroke systems of care: a policy statement from the American Heart Association/American Stroke Association. *Stroke* 2013; 44: 2961–2984. doi:10.1161/STR.0b013e3182a6d2b2.

4. Brainin M, Olsen TS, Chamorro A, *et al*. Organization of stroke care: education, referral, emergency management and imaging, stroke units and rehabilitation. European Stroke Initiative. *Cerebrovasc Dis* 2004; 17 (Suppl 2): 1–14.

5. Hack W, Kaste M, Bogousslavsky J, *et al*. European Stroke Initiative Recommendations for Stroke Management: update 2003. *Cerebrovasc Dis* 2003; 16: 311–337.

6. Kobayashi A, Czlonkowska A, Ford GA, *et al*. European Academy of Neurology and European Stroke Organization consensus statement and practical guidance for

pre-hospital management of stroke. *Eur J Neurol* 2018; 25: 425–433. doi:10.1111/ene.13539.

7. Kim JT, Fonarow GC, Smith EE, *et al*. Treatment with tissue plasminogen activator in the golden hour and the shape of the 4.5-hour time-benefit curve in the national United States Get With The Guidelines-Stroke population. *Circulation* 2017; 135: 128–139. doi:10.1161/CIRCULATIONAHA.116.023336.

8. Menon BK, Sajobi TT, Zhang Y, *et al*. Analysis of workflow and time to treatment on thrombectomy outcome in the Endovascular Treatment for Small Core and Proximal Occlusion Ischemic Stroke (ESCAPE) randomized, controlled trial. *Circulation* 2016; 133: 2279–2286. doi:10.1161/CIRCULATIONAHA.115.019983.

9. Adeoye O, Hornung R, Khatri P, *et al*. Recombinant tissue-type plasminogen activator use for ischemic stroke in the United States: a doubling of treatment rates over the course of 5 years. *Stroke* 2011; 42: 1952–1955. doi:10.1161/STROKEAHA.110.612358.

10. Scholten N, Pfaff H, Lehmann HC, *et al*. [Thrombolysis for acute stroke: a nationwide analysis of regional medical care.] *Fortschr Neurol Psychiatr* 2013; 81: 579–585. doi:10.1055/s-0033-1350496.

11. Schwamm LH, Ali SF, Reeves MJ, *et al*. Temporal trends in patient characteristics and treatment with intravenous thrombolysis among acute ischemic stroke patients at Get With The Guidelines-Stroke hospitals. *Circ Cardiovasc Qual Outcomes* 2013; 6: 543–549. doi:10.1161/CIRCOUTCOMES.111.000303.

12. Morgenstern LB, Staub L, Chan W, *et al*. Improving delivery of acute stroke therapy: the TLL Temple Foundation Stroke Project. *Stroke* 2002; 33: 160–166.

13. Williams O, DeSorbo A, Noble J, *et al*. Child-mediated stroke communication: findings from Hip Hop Stroke. *Stroke* 2012; 43: 163–169. doi:10.1161/STROKEAHA.111.621029.

14. Boden-Albala B, Stillman J, Roberts ET, *et al*. Comparison of acute stroke preparedness strategies to decrease emergency department arrival time in a multiethnic cohort: the Stroke Warning Information and Faster Treatment study. *Stroke* 2015; 46: 1806–1812. doi:10.1161/STROKEAHA.114.008802.

15. Walter S, Kostopoulos P, Haas A, *et al*. Diagnosis and treatment of patients with stroke in a mobile stroke unit versus in hospital: a randomised controlled trial. *Lancet Neurol* 2012; 11: 397–404. doi:10.1016/S1474-4422(12)70057-1.

16. Parker SA, Bowry R, Wu TC, *et al*. Establishing the first mobile stroke unit in the United States. *Stroke* 2015; 46: 1384–1391. doi:10.1161/STROKEAHA.114.007993.

17. Beume LA, Hieber, M, Kaller CP, *et al*. Large vessel occlusion in acute stroke: cortical symptoms are more sensitive prehospital indicators than motor deficits. *Stroke* 2018; 49: 2323–2329. doi:10.1161/STROKEAHA.118.022253.

18. Singer OC, Dvorak F, du Mesnil de Rochemont R, *et al.* A simple 3-item stroke scale: comparison with the National Institutes of Health stroke scale and prediction of middle cerebral artery occlusion. *Stroke* 2005; 36: 773–776. doi:10.1161/01. STR.0000157591.61322.df.

19. Katz BS, McMullan JT, Sucharew H, Adeoye O, Broderick JP. Design and validation of a prehospital scale to predict stroke severity: Cincinnati Prehospital Stroke Severity Scale. *Stroke* 2015; 46: 1508–1512. doi:10.1161/STROKEAHA.115.008804.

20. Lima FO, Silva GS, Furie KL, *et al.* Field assessment stroke triage for emergency destination: a simple and accurate prehospital scale to detect large vessel occlusion strokes. *Stroke* 2016; 47: 1997–2002. doi:10.1161/STROKEAHA.116.013301.

21. Noorian AR, Sanossian N, Shkikova K, *et al.* Los Angeles Motor Scale to indentify large vessel occlusion: prehospital validation and comparison with other screens. *Stroke* 2018; 49: 565–572. doi:10.1161/STROKEAHA.117.019228.

22. Pérez de la Ossa N, Carrera D, Gorchs M, *et al.* Design and validation of a prehospital stroke scale to predict large arterial occlusion: the rapid arterial occlusion evaluation scale. *Stroke* 2014; 45: 87–91.

23. Hastrup S, Damgaard D, Johnsen SP, Andersen G. Prehospital acute stroke severity scale to predict large artery occlusion: design and comparison with other scales. *Stroke* 2016; 47: 1772–1776. doi:10.1161/STROKEAHA.115.012482.

24. Teleb MS, Ver Hage A, Carter J, Jayaraman MV, McTaggart RA. Stroke vision, aphasia, neglect (VAN) assessment: a novel emergent large vessel occlusion screening tool: pilot study and comparison with current clinical severity indices. *J Neurointerv Surg* 2017; 9: 122–126. doi:10.1136/neurintsurg-2015-012131.

25. Ali A, Zachrison KS, Eschenfeldt PC, *et al.* Optimization of prehospital triage of patients with suspected ischemic stroke: results of a mathematical model. *Stroke* 2018; 49: 2532–2535. doi:10.1161/STROKEAHA.118.022041.

26. Holodinsky JK, Williamson TS, Kamal N, *et al.* Drip and ship versus direct to comprehensive stroke center: conditional probability modeling. *Stroke* 2017; 48: 233–238. doi:10.1161/STROKEAHA.116.014306.

27. Direct transfer to an endovascular center compared to transfer to the closest stroke center in acute stroke patients with suspected large vessel occlusion (RACECAT). *ClinicalTrials.gov.* https://clinicaltrials.gov/ct2/show/NCT02795962 (accessed June 2019).

28. Alberts MJ, Hademenos G, Latchaw RE, *et al.* Recommendations for the establishment of primary stroke centers. Brain Attack Coalition. *JAMA* 2000; 283: 3102–3109.

29. The Joint Commission, American Heart Association, American Stroke Association. Primary stroke center certification: overview sheet. www.heart.org/idc/groups/heart-

public/@wcm/@hcm/@ml/documents/downloadable/ucm_455522.pdf (accessed June 2019).

30. Meyer BC, Raman R, Hemmen T, *et al.* Efficacy of site-independent telemedicine in the STRokE DOC trial: a randomised, blinded, prospective study. *Lancet Neurol* 2008; 7: 787–795.

31. Amorim E, Shih M-M, Koehler SA, *et al.* Impact of telemedicine implementation in thrombolytic use for acute ischemic stroke: the University of Pittsburgh Medical Center telestroke network experience. *J Stroke Cerebrovasc Dis* 2013; 22: 527–531.

32. Kepplinger J, Barlinn K, Deckert S, *et al.* Safety and efficacy of thrombolysis in telestroke: a systematic review and meta-analysis. *Neurology* 2016; 87: 1344–1351.

33. Stroke Unit Trialists' Collaboration. Organised inpatient (stroke unit) care for stroke. *Cochrane Database Syst Rev* 2013; (9): CD000197. doi: 10.1002/14651858.CD000197.pub3.

15

Stroke Rehabilitation

Stroke rehabilitation begins during the acute hospitalization once the patient is medically and neurologically stable. Rehabilitation, with involvement of a multidisciplinary rehabilitation team early during the care of the stroke patient, is one of the critical components of stroke unit care that results in improved outcome and shortened length of stay. While practices vary between countries and among hospitals, at our centers and in most US stroke centers the major focus of rehabilitative efforts occurs after discharge from the acute stroke unit, and is beyond the scope of this book (e.g. the EXCITE trial of constraint-induced movement therapy[1]). We will focus on those aspects of rehabilitation care that are relevant to acute stroke management.

The primary goals of acute stroke rehabilitation are to prevent medical complications, minimize impairments, and maximize function while preventing recurrent strokes. The principles of rehabilitation are the same in patients with ischemic stroke and in those with intracerebral hemorrhage.

Early involvement of speech, occupational, and physical therapists in the care of patients on stroke units is associated with a decreased risk of medical complications associated with immobility including aspiration pneumonia, urinary tract infections, falls, and pressure ulcers.[2]

■ Early Acute Stroke Rehabilitation Trials

The body of research to support stroke rehabilitation is growing. There are a number of trials of early acute stroke rehabilitation that are relevant to the acute hospital setting.

- **AVERT 2 (phase II) and AVERT (phase III): A Very Early Rehabilitation Trial for stroke.** In the acute stroke setting, very early mobilization (VEM) focused on assisting patients to be upright and out of bed within 24 hours of stroke was shown to be safe in the phase II AVERT trial.[3] However, in the phase III AVERT trial stroke patients who had VEM were *less* likely to be functionally independent (mRS 0–2) at 3 months as compared to usual care.[4,5] There was no difference in mortality or adverse events between the VEM and usual-care rehabilitation groups.

- **FLAME: Fluoxetine for Motor Recovery after Acute Ischemic Stroke.** In the FLAME trial, patients who received fluoxetine 20 mg within 5–10 days of moderate to severe AIS onset had significantly better motor performance than those who received placebo at 90 days even after controlling for post-stroke depression.[6] Fluoxetine was demonstrated to be safe, and the only notable side effect was gastrointestinal upset.

- **FOCUS: Effects of fluoxetine on functional outcomes after acute stroke: a pragmatic, double-blind, randomized, controlled trial.** In the FOCUS trial, AIS patients who received fluoxetine 20 mg within 2–15 days of a moderate-severity stroke had no difference in functional independence as measured by mRS score at 6 months as compared to placebo.[7] The fluoxetine-treated group were significantly less likely to develop depression, but more likely to suffer bone fractures than the placebo-treated group during the first 6 months post stroke. Motor performance score was not measured.

TAKE-HOME MESSAGES

Rehabilitation priorities on the stroke unit:

- Prevention of medical complications.
- Early assessment of rehabilitation needs, utilizing a multidisciplinary rehabilitation team.
- Early initiation of rehabilitation therapies within 24 hours of stroke may be safe, but has not been shown to improve 3-month outcomes. Increase intensity of therapy, as tolerated by the patient.
- Use of fluoxetine should be individualized in those with depressive symptoms post stroke, and not used routinely for all patients with motor impairments.

■ Multidisciplinary Rehabilitation Team

The main components of the rehabilitation team are speech therapy, physical therapy, occupational therapy, and psychosocial therapy.

SPEECH THERAPY

Speech therapy (ST) in the stroke unit has two main components: assessment of swallowing and assessment of language function. Both are assessed by a speech and language pathologist (SLP).

Swallowing

The need for swallowing assessment has already been addressed in describing the routine care of the patient with infarct and hemorrhage (Chapter 3). Dysphagia (difficulty with swallowing) is common, occurring in 30–65% of post-stroke patients.[8]

Dysphagia may cause malnutrition, dehydration, and aspiration pneumonia. A bedside swallowing screen should be carried out in all patients before allowing them to eat. If patients are unable to swallow effectively within 12–24 hours, a nasogastric tube (NGT) or Dobhoff tube (DHT) should be placed for enteral feeding. In fully conscious patients with hemispheric stroke, generally, this can be removed and the patient fed by mouth within several days. If there is any question, a modified barium swallow (MBS) or a fiberoptic endoscopic evaluation of swallowing (FEES) should be completed to assess for aspiration and the patient's ability to safely swallow food and liquids of varying consistencies.

However, many stroke patients have prolonged dysphagia. Most often this occurs in patients with brainstem strokes or with hemispheric stroke associated with depressed level of consciousness, dementia, or confusion. In these cases, a percutaneous endoscopic gastrostomy (PEG) tube may need to be placed. Generally, we wait 3–5 days or so after the stroke before deciding to place a PEG, though in patients who will obviously need one, there is no reason to wait. Begin the process of planning for a PEG early, since it takes several days to arrange. Antiplatelet or anticoagulation therapy will raise concerns of bleeding risk and should be addressed as early as possible so as not to delay PEG placement. In our hospitals, the procedure can be done by gastroenterologists, general surgeons, or interventional radiologists.

Language

A description of the different aphasic syndromes is beyond the scope of this book. Most stroke patients have non-fluent-type aphasias, where their speech output is reduced or absent, with comprehension being variably affected. It is less common to see pure fluent aphasias affecting only comprehension, though this certainly can occur. Aphasia, especially impaired comprehension, can seriously impede other aspects of rehabilitation since the patient often cannot understand the instructions given by the therapist. As with other aspects of stroke recovery, practice and time with ST will result in at least some improvement in language function, with comprehension usually improving first. Pharmacotherapy with amphetamines or cholinergic and dopaminergic agents may provide benefit for particular aphasic syndromes but is unproven.

The patient's and the family's frustration with impaired ability to communicate should be dealt with in a supportive manner until improvement begins to occur.

PHYSICAL THERAPY

Physical therapy (PT) focuses on bed mobility, transfers, balance, gait training, training to regain normal movement patterns, and wheelchair mobility. Generally, gait training is not begun in earnest until the patient moves off the stroke unit and onto the rehabilitation unit.

In the first few hours after stroke, especially if the patient is fluctuating, we recommend bed rest, keeping the head no higher than 15–30 degrees in order to optimize cerebral perfusion. At the same time, mobilization is important to prevent deconditioning and deep venous thrombosis. Therefore, we often qualify the bed rest order to allow the patient up with physical therapy and nursing attendance. When the patient first gets up in these cases, the physical therapist and nurse should be instructed to measure the blood pressure before and after sitting and standing, and to maintain careful neurological monitoring, to be sure that the blood pressure doesn't fall or the patient deteriorate.

In the stroke unit, the day following admission, the physical therapist will begin to deal with sitting and transferring from bed to chair, and then standing by the bedside. It is important to remember that patients may have impaired balance and generalized weakness, even if they don't demonstrate a hemiparesis or other signs of weakness or ataxia when lying in bed. Therefore, every stroke patient should be considered a fall risk when he or she first gets out of bed, and should not be allowed up unassisted until evaluated by PT. This is for several reasons. Even a day or two lying in bed can result in a general deconditioning that can lead to generalized weakness and orthostatic hypotension. This can be aggravated by antihypertensive and other medications that are well tolerated when the patient is lying flat, but can cause orthostatic changes when the patient gets out of bed. Eighty percent of stroke patients will eventually regain their ability to walk independently, so that tempered optimism is a reasonable approach when dealing with patients and families in the first few days, even in the case of those with hemiplegia.

OCCUPATIONAL THERAPY

Occupational therapy (OT) focuses on fine and gross motor coordination (pinch, opposition, finger to nose, rapid alternating movements), strength (active range of motion, passive range of motion), tone, sensation, activities of daily living (grooming, bathing, upper-extremity dressing, lower-extremity dressing, commode transfer, toileting) and training to regain normal movement patterns. Various assistive devices such as braces and splints may be used to help with supporting weak limbs, stabilizing joints, and avoiding contractures and pressure sores caused by spasticity and immobility. Larger more easily grasped appliances can be used to augment the functional use of a weak limb. The use of these devices is beyond the scope of this chapter.

An important principle of OT is compensation versus facilitation. Put simply, compensation refers to training the unaffected limb to compensate by carrying out functions of the impaired limb, while facilitation refers to repetitive use of the affected limb in order to accelerate recovery and avoid "learned non-use" that might result from over-compensatory reliance on the unaffected limb. Recent animal and human brain-mapping studies have shown unexpected cortical plasticity in areas adjacent to the stroke, and even contralateral brain areas, in response to repeated attempts to move an affected limb or digit or, in the case of an aphasic patient, to talk. The observation of increased metabolic activity in these areas not normally associated with the function of the affected limb or language has stimulated renewed interest in early and intensive rehabilitation efforts.

PSYCHOSOCIAL THERAPY

Psychosocial evaluation during the transition to outpatient care is covered in Chapter 16. The most pressing psychosocial issues to consider in the first few days after stroke onset concern the management of either confusion/delirium or decreased level of arousal.

Delirium

Management of the confused and delirious patient with choice of sedating drugs has been addressed in Chapter 7.

Basic rules:

- Lights on and window shades open during the day.
- Minimize nighttime disruptions.
- Sedate only when necessary.
- Avoid benzodiazepines.
- Haloperidol (Haldol) 0.5–4 mg PO or IV every 6 hours, risperidone (Risperdal) 0.5–1 mg PO at bedtime or twice daily, quetiapine (Seroquel) 12.5–50 mg PO once or twice daily, and ziprasidone (Geodon) 10–20 mg IM/PO once or twice daily are probably best.
- Use soft restraints and move to a private room if possible.

Level of Arousal

Decreased level of arousal is commonly seen in large hemispheric strokes, and this often impedes participation in rehabilitation. It is essential to avoid all potentially sedating medications (e.g., clonidine, tramadol, cyclobenzaprine). Selected patients may benefit from activating or stimulant drugs. Pharmacotherapy is usually not initiated before 1 week post stroke. It is important to be sure that the patient is not sleepy due to metabolic abnormalities or increased ICP (see Chapter 7).

- **Amantadine (Symmetrel)**
  - Dosage: 100 mg morning and noon (initial).
  - Contraindications: epilepsy, any seizure disorder, congestive heart failure or accumulation of fluid (swelling) in arms, legs, hands, or feet, kidney disease, liver disease, chronic rash such as eczema.
  - Side effects: headache, nausea or decreased appetite, depression, anxiety or confusion, insomnia, nervousness, dizziness, lightheadedness, drowsiness, dry mouth, constipation. Close monitoring if on a diuretic.

- **Mondafinil (Provigil)**
  - Dosage: 100 mg morning (initial).
  - Contraindications: angina, recent MI, cirrhosis, seizures.
  - Side effects: headache, nausea, anxiety, insomnia, nervousness, dizziness.

- **Methylphenidate (Ritalin)**
  - Dosage: 5 mg morning and noon (initial).
  - Contraindications: marked anxiety, tension, and agitation, patients with glaucoma, seizures, motor tics, not in combination with a monoamine oxidase inhibitor.
  - Side effects: anxiety, insomnia, nervousness, hypersensitivity reactions, anorexia, dizziness, palpitations, blood-pressure alterations, cardiac arrhythmias.
  - Serious adverse events reported with concomitant use with clonidine.

- **Bromocriptine (Parlodel)**
  - Dosage: 1.25 mg morning and noon (initial).
  - Contraindication: uncontrolled hypertension.
  - Side effects: nausea, headache, dizziness, fatigue, vomiting, drowsiness.

■ Discharge Disposition

Patients will either go home or be transferred to long-term acute care, inpatient rehabilitation, a skilled nursing facility, or a nursing home. This should be determined after evaluating the patient's short- and long-term rehabilitation potential in conjunction with the rehabilitation team, and discussions with the patient and family over resources, home support and environment, and preferred location.

HOME

For the patient who is independent. Consider home safety evaluation, supervision level, and arrange outpatient rehabilitation services if needed.

LONG-TERM ACUTE CARE (LTAC)

For the patient who has medical needs requiring long-term hospitalization, usually for more than a month. An example would be a patient with pneumonia after a tracheostomy and PEG, or patients with other critical-care or medical needs that make them too sick for an inpatient rehabilitation unit or a nursing facility because daily medical care is needed.

INPATIENT REHABILITATION

Rehabilitation completed during an inpatient stay in a rehabilitation unit of an acute care hospital, or in a free-standing rehabilitation hospital. For patients who have good rehabilitation potential but who are not yet able to function independently at home. Must be alert, cooperative, and strong enough to be able to participate in 3 hours of PT and OT daily. Medicare criteria are that patients must be able to tolerate 3 hours of therapy daily, and must require two modalities of therapy, of which one is PT. Usually lasts for 2 weeks.

SKILLED NURSING FACILITY (SNF)

Rehabilitation performed during a stay in a nursing facility, also called "subacute rehabilitation" in some areas. For patients at a lower level than inpatient rehabilitation, these are patients who are not yet able to function independently at home, and can't participate in 3 hours of therapy daily, but do have the potential for improving to that point over the next few months. These patients must be medically stable. If needed, tracheostomy and PEG should be done before transfer. Nursing facilities vary widely in the delivery of rehabilitation services, from limited services to the complete range of rehabilitation services (OT, PT, ST).

NURSING HOME

For patients who are dependent for most of their daily needs, and likely to stay that way. These patients must be medically stable. Usually a PEG does not exclude a patient, but a tracheostomy and the need for frequent suctioning means the patient will need an SNF.

References

1. Wolf SL, Winstein CJ, Miller JP, *et al.*; EXCITE Investigators. Effect of constraint-induced movement therapy on upper extremity function 3 to 9 months after stroke: the EXCITE randomized clinical trial. *JAMA* 2006; 296: 2095–2104. doi:10.1001/jama.296.17.2095.
2. Govan L, Langhorne P, Weir CJ; Stroke Unit Trialists Collaboration. Does the prevention of complications explain the survival benefit of organized inpatient (stroke unit) care? Further analysis of a systematic review. *Stroke* 2007; 38: 2536–2540.

3. Bernhardt J, Dewey H, Thrift A, *et al.* A very early rehabilitation trial for stroke (AVERT): phase II safety and feasibility. *Stroke* 2008; 39: 390–396. doi:10.1161/STROKEAHA.107.492363.

4. AVERT Trial Collaboration group. Efficacy and safety of very early mobilization within 24 h of stroke onset (AVERT): a randomised controlled trial. *Lancet* 2015: 386: 46–55.

5. Langhorne P, Wu O, Rodgers H, Ashburn A, Bernhardt J. A Very Early Rehabilitation Trial after stroke (AVERT): a phase III, multicentre, randomised controlled trial. *Health Technol Assess* 2017; 21: 1–120. doi:10.3310/hta21540.

6. Chollet F, Tardy J, Albucher JF, *et al.* Fluoxetine for motor recovery after acute ischaemic stroke (FLAME): a randomised placebo-controlled trial. *Lancet Neurol* 2011; 10: 123–130. doi:10.1016/S1474-4422(10)70314-8.

7. FOCUS Trial Collaboration. Effects of fluoxetine on functional outcomes after acute stroke (FOCUS): a pragmatic, double-blind, randomised, controlled trial. *Lancet* 2019; 393: 265–274. doi:10.1016/S0140-6736(18)32823-X.

8. Duncan PW, Zorowitz R, Bates B, *et al.* Management of adult stroke rehabilitation care: a clinical practice guideline. *Stroke* 2005; 36: e100–143.

16

Transition to Outpatient Stroke Care

■ Psychosocial Evaluation

It is never too early to begin to educate the patient and family about lifestyle changes and medical treatments to prevent another stroke. These need to be reinforced throughout the hospital and rehabilitation stay, and in the outpatient stroke clinic.

After a major stroke, both the family and the patient go through a grief reaction that at first includes denial and disbelief, and sometimes anger. In particular, the need to insert a PEG is often a crisis point when the family finally comes to terms with the severe disability and prolonged recovery that lies ahead. At this stage, which is usually when the patient is in the acute stroke unit, mainly supportive measures are indicated. More detailed teaching and coping with the consequences of the disability usually wait until after the acute stroke stay, when the realities of the impairment become clearer, and the shock, disorientation, and confusion have worn off. Even in patients fully recovering from their stroke, the threat of another event and the realization of vulnerability usually cause significant emotional consequences.

All members of the multidisciplinary stroke team should be involved in assisting the stroke patient and the family through this major life event. Having a dedicated transitions-of-care coordinator, with a nursing or social-work background, is exceptionally helpful in transitioning from the hospital to the community setting.

■ Stroke Prevention Clinics

Ensuring close follow-up in an outpatient stroke clinic may help ease the transition to the community setting and address the challenges that inevitably arise, as stroke is a major life event. The most common post-stroke sequelae that we see in our stroke clinics are depression, cognitive impairment, and fatigue. A nurse-practitioner-led early stroke clinic follow-up program in North Carolina has been associated with lower 30-day readmissions.[1] Care in stroke prevention clinics in Ontario was more likely to be guideline-based and demonstrated a 26% decreased risk of mortality.[2]

■ Common Post-Stroke Sequelae

- Depression
- Cognitive impairment
- Fatigue

DEPRESSION

Depression in the patient and caregiver is common after stroke. At least 30% of stroke patients suffer from depression within the first year, with a cumulative incidence of 50% at 5 years.[3,4] Incontinence is an important contributor to depression and dependence, in addition to the obvious other causes (paralysis, inability to talk, and pain). Premorbid depressive tendencies are often amplified after a stroke, so that even patients with little disability may become depressed. Stroke location may also play a role, with more depression reported in non-dominant frontal lesions. Post-stroke depression (PSD) is associated with higher morbidity and risk of stroke recurrence. SSRIs may be helpful in the prevention and treatment of PSD to reduce morbidity and mortality.[5]

COGNITIVE IMPAIRMENT

Cognitive impairment affects at least 30% of stroke patients at 3 months, with even minor stroke survivors being affected.[6] Cognitive impairment can significantly impact return to work, activities of daily living at home, and ability to drive. There may be some limited benefit to the use of donepezil in treating post-stroke cognitive impairment.[7,8] At our centers, memory strategies provided by our outpatient SLP and OT providers are often the most helpful intervention in cases of post-stroke cognitive impairment.

FATIGUE

Fatigue is an under-studied sequela of stroke that affects at least 50% of patients.[9] It seems to be independent of depression and its mechanism is not yet well understood. Although treatment of concomitant depression and encouraging physical exercise are common strategies suggested by clinicians, there is no specific medication or intervention proven to alleviate post-stroke fatigue.[10]

References

1. Condon C, Lycan S, Duncan P, *et al*. Reducing readmissions after stroke with a structured nurse practitioner/registered nurse transitional stroke program. *Stroke* 2016; 47: 1599–604. doi:10.1161/STROKEAHA.115.012524.

2. Webster F, Saposnik G, Kapral MK, *et al.* Organized outpatient care: stroke prevention clinic referrals are associated with reduced mortality after transient ischemic attack and ischemic stroke. *Stroke* 2011; 42: 3176–3182.

3. Hackett ML, Pickles K. Part I: frequency of depression after stroke: an updated systematic review and meta-analysis of observational studies. *Int J Stroke* 2014; 9: 1017–1025.

4. Ayerbe L, Ayis S, Wolfe CD, Rudd AG. Natural history, predictors and outcomes of depression after stroke: systematic review and meta-analysis. *Br J Psychiatry* 2013; 202: 14–21.

5. Jorge RE, Robinson RG, Arndt S, *et al.* Mortality and poststroke depression: a placebo-controlled trial of antidepressants. *Am J Psychiatry* 2003; 160: 1823–1829.

6. del Ser T, Barba R, Morin MM, *et al.* Evolution of cognitive impairment after stroke and risk factors for delayed progression. *Stroke* 2005; 36: 2670–2675.

7. Rockwood K, Mitnitski A, Black SE, *et al.* Cognitive change in donepezil treated patients with vascular or mixed dementia. *Can J Neurol Sci* 2013; 40: 564–571.

8. Chang WH, Park YH, Ohn SH, *et al.* Neural correlates of donepezil-induced cognitive improvement in patients with right hemisphere stroke: a pilot study. *Neuropsychol Rehabil* 2011; 21: 502–514.

9. Cumming TB, Packer M, Kramer SF, *et al.* The prevalence of fatigue after stroke: a systematic review and meta-analysis. *Int J Stroke* 2016; 11: 968–977.

10. Wu S, Kutlubaev MA, Chun HY, *et al.* Interventions for post-stroke fatigue. *Cochrane Database Syst Rev* 2015; (7): CD007030.

Appendix 1
IV tPA Dosing Chart

Patient weight		tPA dose (mg)		
			Bolus	**Infusion**
Pounds	**Kilograms**	**Total**	**Over 1 minute**	**Over 1 hour**
99 lb	45 kg	41	4.1	37
101 lb	46 kg	41	4.1	37
104 lb	47 kg	42	4.2	38
106 lb	48 kg	43	4.3	39
108 lb	49 kg	44	4.4	40
110 lb	50 kg	45	4.5	41
112 lb	51 kg	46	4.6	41
115 lb	52 kg	47	4.7	42
117 lb	53 kg	48	4.8	43
119 lb	54 kg	49	4.9	44
121 lb	55 kg	50	5.0	45
123 lb	56 kg	50	5.0	45
126 lb	57 kg	51	5.1	46
128 lb	58 kg	52	5.2	47
130 lb	59 kg	53	5.3	48
132 lb	60 kg	54	5.4	49
134 lb	61 kg	55	5.5	50

(cont.)

Patient weight		tPA dose (mg)		
Pounds	Kilograms	Total	Bolus Over 1 minute	Infusion Over 1 hour
137 lb	62 kg	56	5.6	50
139 lb	63 kg	57	5.7	51
141 lb	64 kg	58	5.8	52
143 lb	65 kg	59	5.9	53
146 lb	66 kg	59	5.9	53
148 lb	67 kg	60	6.0	54
150 lb	68 kg	61	6.1	55
152 lb	69 kg	62	6.2	56
154 lb	70 kg	63	6.3	57
157 lb	71 kg	64	6.4	58
159 lb	72 kg	65	6.5	59
161 lb	73 kg	66	6.6	59
163 lb	74 kg	67	6.7	60
165 lb	75 kg	68	6.8	61
168 lb	76 kg	68	6.8	61
170 lb	77 kg	69	6.9	62
172 lb	78 kg	70	7.0	63
174 lb	79 kg	71	7.1	64
176 lb	80 kg	72	7.2	65
179 lb	81 kg	73	7.3	66
181 lb	82 kg	74	7.4	67
183 lb	83 kg	75	7.5	68
185 lb	84 kg	76	7.6	68
187 lb	85 kg	77	7.7	69
190 lb	86 kg	77	7.7	69
192 lb	87 kg	78	7.8	70
194 lb	88 kg	79	7.9	71
196 lb	89 kg	80	8.0	72
198 lb	90 kg	81	8.1	73
201 lb	91 kg	82	8.2	74
203 lb	92 kg	83	8.3	75
205 lb	93 kg	84	8.4	76

(cont.)

Patient weight		tPA dose (mg)		
			Bolus	**Infusion**
Pounds	**Kilograms**	**Total**	**Over 1 minute**	**Over 1 hour**
207 lb	94 kg	85	8.5	77
209 lb	95 kg	86	8.6	77
212 lb	96 kg	86	8.6	77
214 lb	97 kg	87	8.7	78
216 lb	98 kg	88	8.8	79
218 lb	99 kg	89	8.9	80
≥ 220 lb	≥ 100 kg	90	9.0	81

Patients weighing more than 100 kg (220 lb) receive 90 mg (9 mg bolus and 81 mg infusion).

Appendix 2
Transcranial Doppler Ultrasound

There are many uses of transcranial Doppler ultrasound (TCD):

- Diagnosis of intracranial stenosis
- Diagnosis of acute occlusion
- Monitoring of acute thrombolytic therapy
- Vasoreactivity (vascular reserve) with carotid disease
- Emboli monitoring
- Vascular monitoring during surgery
- Detection of right-to-left shunt (RLS) (most commonly patent foramen ovale)

For the various uses of TCD in stroke refer to Alexandrov, *Cerebrovascular Ultrasound in Stroke Prevention and Treatment* (2011).[1] Here we focus on the detection of RLS.

Procedure for Right-to-Left Shunt Detection

Based on European Society of Neurosonology and Cerebral Hemodynamics consensus, 1999.[2,3]

Equipment

- TCD
- two normal saline bottles 15 mL
- two 10 mL syringes
- flexible tubing
- three-way stopcock

Preparation

The patient must be in the supine position, with the arm horizontal. An intravenous catheter (#18) is inserted into an antecubital vein (connected to a 250 mL bottle of physiologic solution by means of a flexible tube to maintain venous access).

The right middle cerebral artery (MCA) is traced by means of TCD (the examination is more sensitive if bilateral monitoring is used).

Procedure

- Two 10 mL (or 20 mL) syringes are prepared: one containing 9 mL of physiologic solution and the other containing 1 mL of air. By means of a three-way stopcock, the contents of both syringes are rapidly mixed until a homogeneous solution is obtained.
- The solution is rapidly injected in bolus form with the patient at rest. Inject with the syringe pointed superiorly so the bubbles aggregate at the top and are injected first.
- The MCA is monitored for 40–60 seconds.
- The procedure is repeated with Valsalva maneuver.
  - The efficacy of the Valsalva maneuver must be ascertained beforehand through the reduction of the systolic flow velocity on MCA by at least one-third.
  - Five seconds after injection of the contrast agent, the examiner orders the patient to begin the Valsalva maneuver, which must last for at least 10 seconds.

Interpretation

The test is deemed positive if the appearance of at least one microbubble (MB) is recorded as a high-intensity transient signal (HITS) on the TCD trace within 40 seconds of terminating the injection; no agreement exists as to a cutoff interval between contrast injection and MB appearance.

Although it takes about 11 seconds for the bubbles to reach the MCA through an intracardiac shunt, and about 14 seconds through an intrapulmonary shunt, a time window cannot differentiate between RLS at the atrial level and RLS at different sites of the vascular system. It is in any case advisable to record the time of appearance of the first MB.

The results of the two sessions (basal and with Valsalva) must be evaluated separately. Repeated testing may increase the sensitivity, and in the event of discrepancies the positive test must be considered.

- No HITS – test negative
- 1–10 HITS – low-grade shunt
- > 10 HITS, but without "curtain" effect – medium-grade shunt
- Curtain effect, seen when the microbubbles are so numerous as to be no longer distinguishable separately – high-grade shunt

With regard to the physiopathological features of the RLS, we define as:

- **Permanent** – a shunt detected in basal conditions
- **Latent** – a shunt detected only with Valsalva

References

1. Alexandrov AV (ed.). *Cerebrovascular Ultrasound in Stroke Prevention and Treatment*, 2nd edn. Hoboken, NJ; Oxford: Wiley, 2011.

2. Angeli S, Del Sette M, Beelke M, Anzola GP, Zanette E. Transcranial Doppler in the diagnosis of cardiac patent foramen ovale. *Neurol Sci* 2001; 22: 353–356.

3. Jauss M, Zanette E. Detection of right-to-left shunt with ultrasound contrast agent and transcranial Doppler sonography. *Cerebrovasc Dis* 2000; 10: 490–496.

Appendix 3
Medical Complications

This appendix deals with the prevention and treatment of deep venous thrombosis, aspiration pneumonia, urinary tract infection, and heparin-induced thrombocytopenia.

The first three of these are common complications in stroke patients. Heparin-induced thrombocytopenia, while not common, is underdiagnosed.

Deep Venous Thrombosis (DVT)

Prevention
- Enoxaparin (Lovenox) 40 mg SC once daily: probably the best choice. In very large patients, consider 30 mg SC every 12 hours.[1]
- Heparin 5000 units SC every 8–12 hours.
- Dalteparin (Fragmin) 5000 units once daily.
- Compressive stockings and sequential compression devices (SCDs).

Diagnosis
- Venous Doppler ultrasound of the lower (and/or upper) extremities.

Treatment

Choice of therapy will need to take into account acuity and volume of stroke, as well as location of DVT (above versus below the knee).[2]

- In small strokes without hemorrhagic transformation, it may be reasonable to start full-dose weight-adjusted heparin. However, in acute and large strokes, and in those with hemorrhagic conversion, full anticoagulation may not be safe. Low-intensity heparin infusion or inferior vena cava (IVC) filter placement may be suitable alternatives in these cases.
- Above-the-knee DVTs have a higher risk of propagating and causing pulmonary embolism (PE), and therefore these are the DVTs that unequivocally need intervention or treatment.
- The treatment of below-the-knee DVTs draws less consensus. Some will choose to treat while others will observe with serial weekly or biweekly Doppler ultrasounds to monitor for proximal extension of the clot.

Aspiration Pneumonia

Community aspiration pneumonia is usually caused by a mixture of anaerobic organisms, while hospital-acquired aspiration pneumonia is often caused by aerobic organisms (Gram-positive and Gram-negative).

Prevention

- NPO until speech pathology evaluation or bedside evaluation by specially trained nurses.
- Follow speech pathology recommendations.
- Head of bed up.
- Sit upright when eating.
- Assistance with feeding.

Diagnosis

- A constellation of symptoms and signs: fever, hypoxia, chest x-ray infiltrate, leukocytosis, clinical aspiration.

- Sputum culture not very reliable.
- Pneumonia in stroke patients can also occur from bacterial translocation due to a leaky gut–blood barrier rather than aspiration, be it microscopic or frank.

Treatment

- No need to cover for anaerobes, unless severe periodontal disease, necrotizing pneumonia, or lung abscess is present.
- Cover for Gram-positive (MRSA in patients with MRSA risk factors) and Gram-negative (*Pseudomonas*, Enterobacteraciae).

Antibiotic Choices

Be sure to check the patient's allergies.

- Although not well studied in aspiration pneumonia, duration of treatment is usually 7 days, unless it is complicated by empyema or cavitation, in which case we recommend extending coverage up to 14 days.

If early in the clinical course of stroke and the risk of multidrug-resistant organisms is low:

- Ceftriaxone (Rocephin) 1–2 g IV once daily.
- Ampicillin/sulbactam (Unasyn) 3 g IV every 6 hours. Renally cleared. Provides anaerobic coverage.
- Levofloxacin (Levaquin) 750 mg IV once daily. Risk of ECG QT interval prolongation. Renally cleared. Low activity against anaerobes.
- Moxifloxacin (Avelox) 400 mg IV once daily. Risk of ECG QT interval prolongation, especially in those with hepatic impairment. There is a reported increase in resistance of anaerobes to moxifloxacin.
- Piperacillin/tazobactam (Zosyn) 3.375–4.5 g IV every 6 hours. Contains high sodium and is renally cleared. Provides anaerobic coverage.

For suspected multidrug-resistant pathogens:

- For *Pseudomonas* coverage:

- Penicillins/cephalosporins: cefepime (Maxipime) 1–2 g IV every 8–12 hours, ceftazidime 2 g IV every 8 hours, or piperacillin/tazobactam. They are renally cleared.
- Aztreonam is a non-penicillin/cephalosporin alternative.
- Levofloxacin or moxifloxacin, or aminoglycosides (gentamicin or tobramycin 7 mg/kg IV per day carefully dosed).
- For MRSA coverage: vancomycin (Vancocin) 1 g IV every 12 hours (check trough levels before third or fourth dose. Target 10–20 µg/mL). Alternative is linezolid 600 mg IV twice daily.
- For MSSA coverage: nafcillin (Nallpen) 0.5–2 g every 4 hours is better. Cefepime has fair coverage.
- For anaerobic coverage in cases of severe periodontal disease, necrotizing pneumonia, or lung abscess:
  - Clindamycin 600 mg IV twice daily, then later 300 mg PO four times daily.
  - Metronidazole 500 mg PO or IV three times daily plus amoxicillin 500 mg PO three times daily.

Catheter-Associated Urinary Tract Infection (UTI)

Prevention
- Remove indwelling catheter as soon as possible!

Diagnosis
- White blood cells in urinalysis (i.e., pyuria).
- Urine culture of single species > 10^5 (i.e., significant bacteriuria).

Treatment
- Remove or change catheter and start an antibiotic. The final choice of antibiotics should be based on culture results:
  - Trimethoprim–sulfamethoxazole double strength (TMP-SMX, Bactrim DS) 1 tablet PO every 12 hours or TMP-SMX suspension

20 mL per nasojejunal (NJ) tube every 12 hours. Watch for possible
drug–drug interaction as TMP-SMX increases warfarin effect!
- Nitrofurantoin (Furadantin, Macrodantin) 50 mg capsule or
  suspension PO or per NJ tube every 6 hours, or Nitrofurantoin SR
  (Macrobid) 100 mg capsule PO every 12 hours.
- Ciprofloxacin at 500 mg PO or 400 mg IV twice a day
- Levofloxacin 250–500 mg PO or IV once daily.
- Piperacillin/tazobactam 3.375 mg IV every 8 hours.
- If *Pseudomonas aeruginosa* is suspected, treatment
  with ciprofloxacin, ceftazidime (1 g IV every 8 hours),
  or cefepime (1 g IV every 12 hours).
- Duration 3–5 days. If this is catheter-associated (i.e., CAUTI), then treat
  for 7–14 days depending on clinical response.
- Check culture for final antibiotic choice.

Heparin-Induced Thrombocytopenia (HIT)

Prevention
- Do not use heparin unless necessary, and check platelet counts daily.

Diagnosis
HIT is underdiagnosed. 5% of patients given unfractionated heparin
develop antibodies and 3% get HIT with thrombotic syndrome (HITTS). It
is more common with intravenous versus subcutaneous use, high dose
versus low dose, unfractionated versus low-molecular-weight heparin
(rare).
- Platelets drop 50% compared with baseline, or < 100 000. Check platelet
  count daily in patients on heparin. Check PF4 antiplatelet antibodies
  and serotonin release assay (SRA) if PF4 immunoassay is indeterminate.
- Clinical consequences include DVT, pulmonary emboli,
  cardioembolism, peripheral vascular occlusion, MI, stroke.

- Consider HITTS in any patient with unexplained thromboembolic event after heparin exposure. Remember, platelet count may not be low – just 50% drop compared with baseline, and baseline may be well above 200 000.
- **Type 1** – transient, mild, starts 4 days after exposure but can start after a longer interval and after heparin is stopped.
- **Type 2** – two types:
  - 4–14 days after exposure
  - < 12 hours after exposure

Treatment

- Stop heparin.
- Even so, 50% will still develop HITTS once platelet count starts to fall if you just stop heparin.
- No warfarin until platelets normalize.
- No platelets.
- Thrombin inhibitor even before platelet antibody test result is back:
  - Argatroban: reversible, more potent, non-antigenic, hepatic clearance. Half-life = 40–50 minutes. Adjust PTT every 2–4 hours to 1.5–3 × control. Start at 2 μg/minute; titrate up to < 10 μg/minute.
  - Lepirudin (Refludan): irreversible, antigenic, renal clearance. Bolus 0.4 mg/kg, then infusion.
  - Bivalirudin (Angiomax) is not approved by FDA or EMA for HIT.

References

1. Hillbom M, Erila T, Sotaniemi K, *et al.* Enoxaparin vs heparin for prevention of deep-vein thrombosis in acute ischaemic stroke: a randomized, double-blind study. *Acta Neurol Scand* 2002; 106: 84–92.
2. Kearon C, Akl EA, Comerota AJ, *et al.* Antithrombotic therapy for VTE disease: Antithrombotic therapy and prevention of thrombosis, 9th ed: American College of Chest Physicians evidence-based clinical practice guidelines. *Chest* 2012; 141 (2 Suppl): e419S–e496S. Erratum in *Chest* 2012; 142: 1698–1704.

Appendix 4
Brainstem Syndromes

The pattern of cranial nerve abnormalities is the key to distinguishing among these.

Lateral Medullary Syndrome

Also known as **Wallenberg syndrome**. The crossed sensory findings, i.e., loss of sensation on one side of the face and the other side of the body, are pathognomonic.

- vertigo, nausea, diplopia
- ipsilateral headache (descending spinal tract of the fifth cranial nerve, facial or eye pain)
- ataxia, hiccups
- contralateral body hemianalgesia (pain + temperature)
- ipsilateral facial hemianalgesia (pain + temperature)
- Horner syndrome, nystagmus
- ipsilateral palate, vocal cord weakness (nucleus ambiguus)
- dysphagia
- cerebellar findings
- motor, tongue function, dorsal column function spared because these structures lie medially in the medulla

- due to occlusion of the ipsilateral vertebral artery or its major branch, the posterior inferior cerebellar artery

Millard–Gubler Syndrome

Ventrocaudal pons with CN VI and VII involvement
- contralateral hemiplegia (pyramidal tract)
- ipsilateral lateral rectus paresis (VI)
- ipsilateral lower motor neuron (LMN) facial paresis (VII)

Foville Syndrome

Dorsal caudal pontine lesion
- contralateral body hemiplegia
- ipsilateral LMN facial paresis (VII)
- inability to move eyes to same side as lesion (parapontine reticular formation, CN VI)

Raymond–Cestan Syndrome

Dorsal rostral pons
- ataxia with coarse tremor
- contralateral hemisensory loss (face + body, all modalities)
- ± contralateral hemiparesis

Marie–Foix Syndrome

Lateral pons
- ipsilateral cerebellar ataxia
- contralateral hemiparesis
- ± contralateral hemisensory loss (pain and temperature) due to spinothalamic tract

Weber Syndrome

Ventral midbrain
- contralateral hemiplegia (corticospinal and corticobulbar tracts)
- ipsilateral oculomotor paresis, dilated pupil

Benedikt Syndrome

Midbrain tegmentum (red nucleus, CN III)
- ipsilateral oculomotor paresis, dilated pupil
- contralateral intention tremor, hemichorea, hemiathetosis

Claude Syndrome

Midbrain tegmentum
- ipsilateral oculomotor paresis
- contralateral cerebellar ataxia

Parinaud Syndrome

Dorsal midbrain (often with hydrocephalus, tumor)
- upgaze paresis
- convergence–retraction nystagmus on upgaze
- large pupil with light-near dissociation, lid retraction, lid lag

Appendix 5
Anatomy of Cerebral Vasculature

Circle of Willis

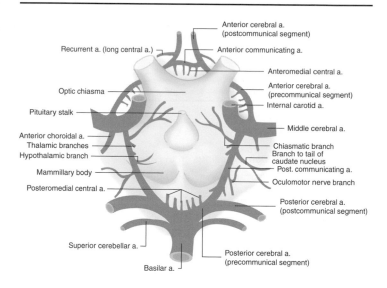

Anterior cerebral a.
(postcommunical segment)

Anterior communicating a.

Recurrent a. (long central a.)

Anteromedial central a.

Optic chiasma

Anterior cerebral a.
(precommunical segment)

Internal carotid a.

Pituitary stalk

Middle cerebral a.

Anterior choroidal a.

Chiasmatic branch

Thalamic branches

Branch to tail of
caudate nucleus

Hypothalamic branch

Post. communicating a.

Mammillary body

Oculomotor nerve branch

Posteromedial central a.

Posterior cerebral a.
(postcommunical segment)

Superior cerebellar a.

Posterior cerebral a.
(precommunical segment)

Basilar a.

Arteries of the Brain

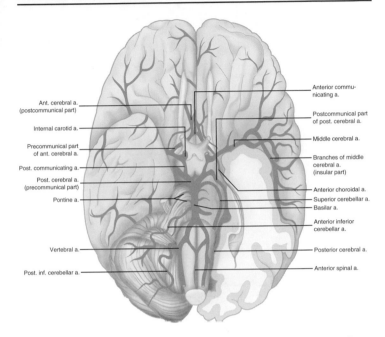

Ant. cerebral a. (postcommunical part)

Internal carotid a.

Precommunical part of ant. cerebral a.

Post. communicating a.

Post. cerebral a. (precommunical part)

Pontine a.

Vertebral a.

Post. inf. cerebellar a.

Anterior communicating a.

Postcommunical part of post. cerebral a.

Middle cerebral a.

Branches of middle cerebral a. (insular part)

Anterior choroidal a.

Superior cerebellar a.

Basilar a.

Anterior inferior cerebellar a.

Posterior cerebral a.

Anterior spinal a.

Arteries at the base of skull (arterial circle of Willis and its branches, basilar artery), inferior (brain) view.

Veins of the Brain

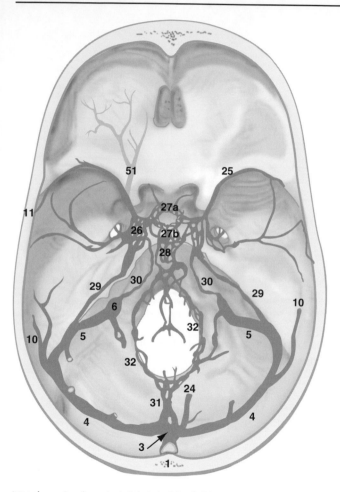

A top-down view (superior to inferior) of the skull base. The venous circulation in the skull base region is visualized. The numerous venous communications that exist around the skull base are also illustrated.

1 superior sagittal sinus

3 torcular Herophili

4 transverse sinus

5 sigmoid sinus

6 jugular bulb

10 vein of Labbé

11 superficial middle cerebral vein

24 straight sinus

25 sphenoparietal sinus

26 cavernous sinus

27a anterior intercavernous sinus

27b posterior intercavernous sinus

28 clival venous plexus

29 superior petrosal sinus

30 inferior petrosal sinus

31 occipital sinus

32 marginal sinus

51 superior ophthalmic vein

Reprinted with permission from the Cleveland Clinic Foundation.

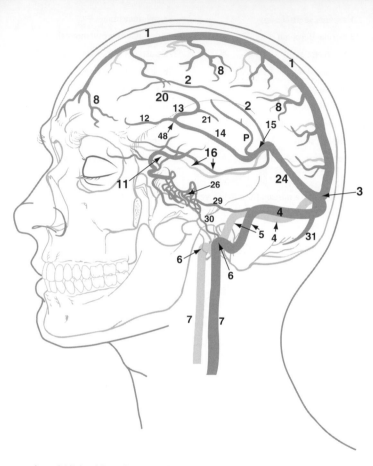

Near-lateral (slight obliquity) view of the supratentorial, superficial, and deep venous systems.

1 superior sagittal sinus
2 inferior sagittal sinus
3 torcular Herophili
4 transverse sinus
5 sigmoid sinus
6 jugular bulb
7 internal jugular vein
8 superficial cortical vein
11 superficial middle cerebral vein
12 septal vein
13 thalamostriate vein

14 internal cerebral vein
15 great cerebral vein of Galen
16 basal vein of Rosenthal
20 anterior caudate vein
21 terminal vein
26 cavernous sinus
29 superior petrosal sinus
30 inferior petrosal sinus
31 occipital sinus
48 true venous angle
P posterior pericallosal vein

Reprinted with permission from the Cleveland Clinic Foundation.

Appendix 6
Brain Death Criteria

According to the US Uniform Determination of Death Act (UDDA), death by neurological criteria is defined as the irreversible loss of the capacity for consciousness combined with the irreversible loss of all brain and brainstem functions, including the capacity to breathe. Institutional diagnostic protocols differ, and there is variability in how many exams are needed, the minimal time lapse between exams, and who can perform a brain death exam. Very crucial to the diagnosis of brain death, nonetheless, is excluding all potential clinical confounders of coma. The following criteria are derived from the 2010 revised American Academy of Neurology practice parameter guidelines.[1]

Nature of Coma Must Be Known

- Known structural disease or irreversible systemic metabolic cause that can explain the clinical picture.

Confounding Causes Must Be Ruled Out

- Body temperature must be above 36 °C.

- No presence of drug intoxication (mostly benzodiazepines, barbiturates, narcotics/opioids) or neuromuscular blockade.
- Patient is not in shock (SBP must be > 100 mmHg).
- No significant metabolic derangements coexist (severe electrolyte disturbances, hepatic or renal failure, acid–base disorders, hyperammonemia, significant endocrine dysfunction).

Absence of Cerebral and Brainstem Function

- No spontaneous movement or eye opening, and no eye, verbal, or motor response to noxious stimulation (i.e., no flexor or extensor posturing).
- Absent pupillary reflex. Make sure pupils were not pharmacologically dilated prior to exam.
- Absent oculocephalic reflex (i.e., doll's eyes). Test is contraindicated in patients with cervical spinal cord injury.
- Absent oculovestibular reflex (i.e., cold calorics). Test is contraindicated in patients with skull-base fractures.
- Absent corneal reflex.
- Absent gag reflex.
- Absent cough reflex.
- Absence of spontaneous or responsive movement to noxious stimulation (e.g., localization, withdrawal, decorticate, or decerebrate). Primitive movements in response to local painful stimuli, mediated at a spinal-cord level, can however occur (i.e., "triple flexion," plantar responses, deep tendon reflexes).
- No spontaneous respirations.
- Some protocols require independent exams 6, 12, or 24 hours apart by a board-eligible or certified neurologist or neurosurgeon.

Apnea Test

- Should only be attempted in the hemodynamically stable patient. Abort if SpO_2 < 85% for > 30 seconds.
- Preoxygenate with 100% O_2 for 5 minutes to PaO_2 > 200 mmHg. $PaCO_2$ should be normalized to 40 ± 5 mmHg.
- Obtain baseline arterial blood gas.
- Disconnect the patient from the ventilator circuit, and give 6 L/minute of 100% O_2 via nasal cannula introduced into the endotracheal tube and lowered to the level of the carina.
- Observe for spontaneous respirations. If hypotension or arrhythmia occurs, immediately reconnect the ventilator, abort the apnea testing, and obtain an ancillary confirmatory test (see below).
- At intervals of 8–10 minutes, draw serial arterial blood gases until $PaCO_2$ rises to 60 mmHg or 20 mmHg above the baseline $PaCO_2$ level.
- Reconnect to ventilator.

Confirmatory Tests

These are not necessary to diagnose brain death. However, some protocols allow the diagnosis of brain death based on these studies.

Therefore, they can be used in situations where it is not quite certain if the criteria are met on the physical exam, and also to bypass the prolonged observation period and the need for repeated testing. Commonly, when the apnea test or a portion of the exam cannot be completed for any reason, an ancillary test will be performed. They are frequently employed in patients who are candidates for organ donation.

- Cerebral blood flow studies with documentation of absent flow on one of the following:
  - conventional angiogram
  - nuclear medicine cerebral blood flow study
- Electroencephalogram (EEG) with no physiologic brain activity.

- Transcranial Doppler (TCD) demonstrating reverberating flow or short systolic spikes but no diastolic flow.

Timing of brain death corresponds to the time the $PaCO_2$ reached the target value or the time the ancillary test was officially interpreted.

References

1. Wijdicks EF, Varelas PN, Gronseth GS, Greer DM; American Academy of Neurology. Evidence-based guideline update: determining brain death in adults: report of the Quality Standards Subcommittee of the American Academy of Neurology. *Neurology* 2010; 74: 1911–1918. doi:10.1212/WNL.0b013e3181e242a8.

Appendix 7
Stroke Assessment Scales

Stroke Prevention and Anticoagulation
- CHA_2DS_2-VASc scale
- HAS-BLED scale

Coma Scale
- Glasgow Coma Scale (GCS)

Hemorrhage Scales
- ICH score
- Hunt and Hess scale for non-traumatic SAH
- World Federation of Neurological Surgeons (WFNS) scale for SAH

Long-Term Outcome Scale
- Modified Rankin scale

Acute Stroke Scale
- National Institutes of Health Stroke Scale (NIHSS)

CHA₂DS₂-VASc Risk Score

The CHA$_2$DS$_2$-VASc score helps determine the 1-year risk for stroke in a non-anticoagulated patient with non-valvular AF.[1]

CHA$_2$DS$_2$-VASc risk criteria	
Age	< 65 years (0 points) 65–74 years (1 point) ≥ 75 years (2 points)
Sex	Female (1 point) Male (0 points)
Congestive heart failure	Present (1 point) Absent (0 points)
Hypertension	Present (1 point) Absent (0 points)
Diabetes mellitus	Present (1 point) Absent (0 points)
Vascular disease (prior MI, peripheral artery disease, or aortic plaque)	Present (1 point) Absent (0 points)
Stroke/TIA/thromboembolism history	Present (2 points) Absent (0 points)

Score	Annual stroke risk (%)
0	0.2
1	0.6
2	2.2
3	3.2
4	4.8
5	7.2
6	9.7
7	11.2
8	10.8

HAS-BLED Score

Estimates risk of major bleeding in patients on anticoagulation and is used to assess risk–benefit ratio of anticoagulation for atrial fibrillation.[2]

Hypertension (uncontrolled or > 160 mmHg systolic)	Present (1 point) Absent (0 point)
Renal disease (dialysis, transplant, Cr > 2.26 mg/dL or > 200 µmol/L)	Present (1 point) Absent (0 point)
Liver disease (cirrhosis or bilirubin > 2× normal with AST/ALT/AP > 3× normal)	Present (1 point) Absent (0 point)
Stroke history	Present (1 point) Absent (0 point)
Prior major bleeding or predisposition to bleeding	Present (1 point) Absent (0 point)
Labile INR (unstable/high INRs, time in therapeutic range < 60%)	Present (1 point) Absent (0 point)
Age > 65	Present (1 point) Absent (0 point)
Medication usage predisposing to bleeding (aspirin, clopidogrel, NSAIDs)	Present (1 point) Absent (0 point)
Alcohol use (≥ 8 drinks/week)	Present (1 point) Absent (0 point)

Score	Risk (%)
0	0.9
1	3.4
2	4.1
3	5.8 (high risk)
4	8.9
5	9.1
≥ 6	Assumed at least 10%

Glasgow Coma Scale (GCS)

This scale is used in assessing depth of coma, and is therefore not useful for most stroke patients.

The scale adds three components (E + M + V) for a total score of 3–15.

Response	Score	Characteristics
E: Eye opening		
None	1	Eyes always closed; not attributable to ocular swelling
To pain	2	Eyes open in response to painful stimulus
To speech	3	Eyes open in response to speech or shout
Spontaneous	4	Eyes open; does not imply intact awareness
M: Best motor response		
No response	1	No motor response to pain
Extension	2	Extension at elbow
Abnormal flexion	3	Includes preceding extension, stereotyped flexion posture, extreme wrist flexion, abduction of upper arm, flexion of fingers over thumb
Withdrawal	4	Normal flexor withdrawal; no localizing attempt to remove stimulus
Localizes pain	5	Attempt made to remove stimulus; e.g., hand moves above chin toward supraocular stimulus
Obeys commands	6	Follows simple commands
V: Best verbal response		
No response	1	No sounds
Incomprehensible	2	Moaning, groaning, grunting; incomprehensible
Inappropriate	3	Intelligible words, but not in a meaningful exchange; e.g., shouting, swearing
Confused	4	Responds to questions in conversational manner, but responses indicate varying degrees of disorientation and confusion
Oriented	5	Normal orientation to time, place, person

Source: Teasdale G, Jennett B. Assessment of coma and impaired consciousness: a practical scale. *Lancet* 1974; 2: 81–84. Reproduced with permission from Elsevier.[3]

ICH Score

For prognosis in patients with intracerebral hemorrhage (ICH). See *ICH Outcome* in Chapter 12.

Component	ICH score points
GCS score	___
3–4	2
5–12	1
13–15	0
ICH volume, mL	___
≥ 30	1
< 30	0
IVH	___
Yes	1
No	0
Infratentorial origin of ICH	___
Yes	1
No	0
Age, years	___
≥ 80	1
< 80	0
Total ICH score (0–6)	___

GCS score: Glasgow coma score on initial presentation (or after resuscitation).

ICH volume: volume on initial CT calculated using ABC/2 method (see Figure 12.2).

IVH: presence of any intraventricular hemorrhage on initial CT.

Source: Hemphill JC, Bonovich DC, Besmertis L, *et al.* The ICH score: a simple, reliable grading scale for intracerebral hemorrhage. *Stroke* 2001; 32: 891–897.[4] Reproduced with permission.

Hunt and Hess Scale for Non-Traumatic SAH

This scale is used for assessing severity and prognosis in patients with subarachnoid hemorrhage (SAH).

Grade	
1	Asymptomatic, mild headache, slight nuchal rigidity
2	Moderate to severe headache, nuchal rigidity
	No neurologic deficit other than CN palsy
3	Drowsiness/confusion
	Mild focal neurologic deficit
4	Stupor
	Moderate to severe hemiparesis
5	Coma
	Decerebrate posturing

Source: Hunt WE, Hess RM. Surgical risk as related to time of intervention in the repair of intracranial aneurysms. *J Neurosurg* 1968; 28: 14–20.[5] Reproduced with permission from the *Journal of Neurosurgery*.

WFNS Scale for SAH

Another scale used in prognosis for SAH. WFNS = World Federation of Neurological Surgeons.

Grade	
1	GCS 15 = good grade
2	GCS 14–13, with no motor deficit = fair grade
3	GCS 14–13, with hemiparesis or aphasia = tending to poor grade
4	GCS 12–8, with or without hemiparesis or aphasia = poor grade
5	GCS < 8, with or without hemiparesis or aphasia = moribund patient

Adapted from: Teasdale GM, Drake CG, Hunt W, *et al.* A universal subarachnoid hemorrhage scale: report of a committee of the World Federation of Neurosurgical Societies. *J Neurol Neurosurg Psychiatry* 1988; 51: 1457.[6] Reproduced with permission from BMJ Publishing Group.

Modified Rankin Scale (mRS)

A scale commonly used to measure disability or dependence in activities of daily living.[7-9]

Score	Description
0	No symptoms at all
1	No significant disability despite symptoms; able to carry out all usual duties and activities
2	Slight disability; unable to carry out all previous activities, but able to look after own affairs without assistance
3	Moderate disability; requiring some help, but able to walk without assistance
4	Moderately severe disability; unable to walk without assistance and unable to attend to own bodily needs without assistance
5	Severe disability; bedridden, incontinent and requiring constant nursing care and attention
6	Dead
Total	(0–6): ___

National Institutes of Health Stroke Scale (NIHSS)

This is the most commonly used scale for assessing the severity of stroke.[10,11] It is most useful for the initial grading of stroke severity and for following its course. It is less useful for determining outcome, since it does not measure function. It has been proven reliable and reproducible, but requires training and certification.

- The NIHSS forms are available from the NIH website at www.stroke.nih.gov.
- The training can be obtained at https://secure.trainingcampus.net/uas/modules/trees/windex.aspx?rx=nihss-english.trainingcampus.net, as well as from other sites.

Guides to scoring to improve consistency:

- Score the first response that the patient makes.

- Score only if abnormality is present for some items (e.g., ataxia is absent if the patient is hemiplegic).
- Record what the patient does, not what you think the patient can do. The pictures at the end of this appendix are used for standardizing the aphasia exam. Have the patient read the words, name the objects, and describe what is happening in the picture.

1a. Level of consciousness (LOC) A 3 is scored only if the patient makes no movement (other than reflexive posturing) in response to noxious stimulation.	0 = Alert: keenly responsive. 1 = Not alert, but arousable by minor stimulation to obey, answer, or respond. 2 = Not alert, obtunded. Requires repeated stimulation to attend, or requires strong or painful stimulation to make movements.	1a: ___
1b. LOC questions Ask the month and his/her age. Aphasic and stuporous patients who do not comprehend the questions → score 2. Endotracheal intubation, severe dysarthria, language barrier and problems other than aphasia → score 1. Grade the initial answer.	0 – Answers both questions correctly. 1 = Answers one question correctly. 2 = Answers neither question correctly.	1b: ___
1c. LOC commands Open and close the eyes. Open and close the non-paretic hand.	0 = Performs both tasks correctly. 1 = Performs one task correctly.	1c: ___

(cont.)

Only the first attempt is scored.

2. Best gaze

Only voluntary or reflexive (oculocephalic) eye movements are tested. Caloric testing is not done.

A conjugate deviation of the eyes that can be overcome by voluntary or reflexive activity → score 1.

Isolated cranial nerve paresis (CN III, IV, or VI) → score 1

Gaze is testable in all aphasic patients.

2 = Performs neither task correctly.

0 = Normal.   2: ___

1 = Partial gaze palsy. Gaze is abnormal in one or both eyes, but forced deviation or total gaze paresis are not present.

2 = Forced deviation, or total gaze paresis not overcome by the oculocephalic maneuver.

3. Visual fields

Both upper and lower quadrants are tested by confrontation, using finger counting.

Unable to make proper response (e.g., aphasia, obtundation) → use blink to visual threat from the side.

Unilateral blindness or enucleation → test in the remaining eye.

0 = No visual loss.   3: ___

1 = Partial hemianopia (e.g., quadrantanopia, extinction to bilateral simultaneous stimulation).

2 = Complete hemianopia.

3 = Bilateral hemianopia (blind, including cortical blindness).

4. Facial palsy

Ask, or use pantomime to encourage the patient to show teeth or raise eyebrows and close eyes.

0 = Normal symmetrical movement.   4: ___

1 = Minor paralysis (flattened nasolabial

(cont.)

Poorly responsive or non-comprehending patient → use symmetry of grimace in response to noxious stimuli.

fold, asymmetry on smiling).

2 = Partial paralysis (total or near total paralysis of lower face).

3 = Complete paralysis of one or both sides (absence of facial movement in the upper and lower face).

5 & 6. Motor arm and leg

The limb is placed in the appropriate position:

Arm extended with palms down 90 degrees (if sitting) or 45 degrees (if supine) for 10 seconds.

Leg extended at 30 degrees (always tested supine) for 5 seconds.

The aphasic patient is encouraged using urgency in the voice and pantomime but not noxious stimulation.

0 = No drift. Limb holds 90 (or 45) degrees for full 10 seconds (arm) or 30 degrees for 5 seconds (leg).

1 = Drift. Limb drifts down before full 10 seconds (arm) or 5 seconds (leg); does not hit bed or other support.

2 = Some effort against gravity. Limb cannot get to or maintain position and drifts down to bed, but has some effort against gravity.

3 = No effort against gravity. Limb falls.

4 = No movement.

9 = Amputation or joint fusion. Do not add to total score. Explain.

5a. Left arm: ___
5b. Right arm: ___
6a. Left leg: ___
6b. Right leg: ___

7. Limb ataxia

The finger–nose–finger and heel–shin tests are

0 = Absent.

1 = Present in one limb.

2 = Present in two limbs.

7: ___

(cont.)

performed on both sides, and ataxia is scored only if present out of proportion to weakness.

In case of visual defect, ensure testing is done in intact visual field.

Ataxia is absent in the patient who cannot understand or is paralyzed.

In case of blindness test by touching nose from extended arm position.

9 = Amputation or joint fusion. Do not add to total score. Explain.

8. Sensory

Sensation or grimace to pinprick, or withdrawal from noxious stimulus in the obtunded or aphasic patient.

Only sensory loss attributed to stroke is scored as abnormal. Test as many body areas (arms [not hands], legs, trunk, face) as needed to be accurate.

Score 2 only when a severe or total loss of sensation can be clearly demonstrated.

Brainstem stroke with bilateral loss of sensation → score 2.

0 = Normal. No sensory loss.

1 = Mild to moderate sensory loss. Patient feels pinprick is less sharp or is dull on the affected side;

or there is a loss of superficial pain with pinprick but patient is aware he/she is being touched.

2 = Severe to total sensory loss. Patient is not aware of being touched in the face, arm, or leg.

8: ___

(cont.)

Patient does not respond
and is quadriplegic →
score 2.
Coma (item 1a = 3) →
score 2.

9. Best language

The patient is asked to
describe what is
happening in the picture,
to name the items on the
naming sheet, and to
read from the list of
sentences.
Comprehension is judged
from responses here as
well as to all of the
commands in the
preceding general
neurological exam.
Visual loss interferes with
the tests → ask patient to
identify objects placed in
the hand, repeat, and
produce speech.
Intubated patient → ask
patient to write
responses.
Coma (item 1a = 3) → score
3.
Give adequate time, but
only the first response is
measured.

0 = No aphasia, normal.   9: ___
1 = Mild to moderate
aphasia. Some obvious
loss of fluency or facility
of comprehension,
without significant
limitation on ideas
expressed or form of
expression.
2 = Severe aphasia. All
communication is
through fragmentary
expression; great need
for inference,
questioning, and
guessing by the listener.
3 = Mute, global aphasia.
No usable speech or
auditory
comprehension.

10. Dysarthria

A sample of speech must be
obtained by asking the
patient to read or repeat

0 = Normal.   10: ___
1 = Mild to moderate. Patient
slurs at least some words
and, at worst, can be

(cont.)

words from the list. If the patient has severe aphasia, the clarity of articulation of spontaneous speech can be rated.

Mute due to aphasia → score 2.

Intubation or physical barrier → do not score.

understood with some difficulty.

2 = Severe. Patient's speech is so slurred as to be unintelligible in the absence of or out of proportion to any dysphasia, or is mute/anarthric.

9 = Intubated or other physical barrier. Do not add to total score. Explain.

11. Extinction and inattention

Sufficient information to identify neglect may be obtained during the prior testing.

Aphasia but appears to attend to both sides → normal.

Since the abnormality is scored only if present, the item is never untestable.

0 = No abnormality.   11: ___

1 = Present. Visual, tactile, auditory, spatial, or personal inattention or extinction to bilateral simultaneous stimulation in one of the sensory modalities.

2 = Profound hemi-inattention or hemi-inattention to more than one modality. Does not recognize own hand or orients to only one side of space.

For the dysarthria exam, have the patient say the following words

MAMA

TIP – TOP

FIFTY – FIFTY

THANKS

HUCKLEBERRY

BASEBALL PLAYER

CATERPILLAR

For the aphasia exam, have the patient name
the objects pictured below

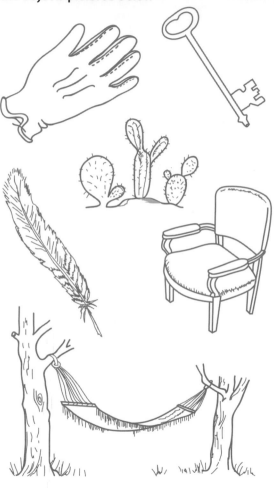

For the aphasia exam, have the patient read the following sentences

You know how.

Down to earth.

I got home from work.

Near the table in the dining room.

They heard him speak on the radio last night.

For the aphasia exam, have the patient describe what is happening in the picture below

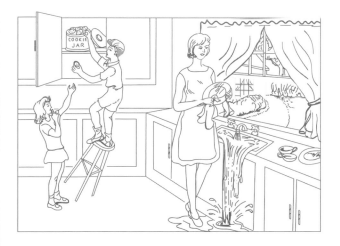

References

1. Pisters R, Lane DA, Nieuwlaat R, *et al.* A novel user-friendly score (HAS-BLED) to assess 1-year risk of major bleeding in patients with atrial fibrillation. *Chest* 2010; 138: 1093–1100. doi:10.1378/chest.10-0134.

2. Lip GY, Nieuwlaat R, Pisters R, *et al.* Refining clinical risk stratification for predicting stroke and thromboembolism in atrial fibrillation using a novel risk factor-based approach: the Euro Heart Survey on Atrial Fibrillation. *Chest* 2010; 137: 263–272. doi:10.1378/chest.09-1584.

3. Teasdale G, Jennett B. Assessment of coma and impaired consciousness: a practical scale. *Lancet* 1974; 2: 81–84.

4. Hemphill JC, Bonovich DC, Besmertis L, Manley GT, Johnston SC. The ICH score: a simple, reliable grading scale for intracerebral hemorrhage. Stroke 2001; 32: 891–897.

5. Hunt WE, Hess RM. Surgical risk as related to time of intervention in the repair of intracranial aneurysms. *J Neurosurg* 1968; 28: 14–20.

6. Teasdale GM, Drake CG, Hunt W, *et al.* A universal subarachnoid hemorrhage scale: report of a committee of the World Federation of Neurosurgical Societies. *J Neurol Neurosurg Psychiatry* 1988; 51: 1457.

7. Rankin J. Cerebral vascular accidents in patients over the age of 60. *Scott Med J* 1957; 2: 200–215.

8. Bonita R, Beaglehole R. Modification of Rankin scale: recovery of motor function after stroke. *Stroke* 1988; 19: 1497–1500.

9. Van Swieten JC, Koudstaal PJ, Visser MC, Schouten HJ, van Gijn J. Interobserver agreement for the assessment of handicap in stroke patients. *Stroke* 1988; 19: 604–607.

10. Goldstein LB, Bertels C, Davis JN. Interrater reliability of the NIH stroke scale. *Arch Neurol* 1989; 46: 660–662.

11. Lyden P, Raman R, Liu L, *et al.* NIHSS training and certification using a new digital video disk is reliable. *Stroke* 2005; 36: 2446–2449.

Further In-Depth Reading

Textbooks

Grotta JC, Albers GW, Broderick JP, *et al.* *Stroke: Pathophysiology, Diagnosis, and Management*, 6th edn. Philadelphia, PA: Elsevier, 2015.

The most comprehensive text on all aspects of stroke pathophysiology, diagnosis, and treatment.

Hankey GJ, Macleod M, Gorelick PB, *et al.* (eds.). *Warlow's Stroke: Practical Management*, 4th edn. Oxford: Wiley-Blackwell, 2019.

A practical textbook that walks the reader through approaching the management of stroke patients using a question-and-answer format.

Caplan LR. *Caplan's Stroke: a Clinical Approach*, 5th edn. Cambridge: Cambridge University Press, 2016.

A clinical guide to stroke care including clinical presentation, causes, evaluation, management, prevention, and recovery.

Caplan LR, van Gijn J. *Stroke Syndromes*, 3rd edn. Cambridge: Cambridge University Press, 2012.

An in-depth reference of clinical presentations of stroke syndromes and their differential diagnosis, aimed at helping clinicians with anatomical localization.

Caplan LR, Biller J. *Uncommon Causes of Stroke*, 3rd edn. Cambridge: Cambridge University Press, 2018.

A detailed guide to the less common causes of stroke, with recently added chapters on stroke in patients with HIV, Lyme disease, and scleroderma.

Roach S, Betterman K, Biller J. *Toole's Cerebrovascular Disorders*, 6th edn. Cambridge: Cambridge University Press, 2010.

An accessible, practical guide to the diagnosis and treatment of stroke.

Lyden PD. *Thrombolytic Therapy for Acute Stroke*, 2nd edn. Totowa, NJ: Humana Press, 2005.

In-depth coverage of all aspects surrounding the use of tPA for acute ischemic stroke.

Guidelines

AHA/ASA scientific statement. Guidelines for the early management of patients with ischemic stroke. *Stroke* 2018; 49: e46–e110.

AHA/ASA science advisory. Expansion of the time window for treatment of acute ischemic stroke with intravenous tissue plasminogen activator. *Stroke* 2009; 40: 2945–2948.

European Stroke Organisation. Guidelines for management of acute ischaemic stroke and spontaneous intracerebral haemorhage. https://eso-stroke.org/eso-guideline-direc tory (accessed June 2019).

AHA/ASA scientific statement. Definition and evaluation of transient ischemic attack. *Stroke* 2009; 40: 2276–2293.

AHA/ASA guideline. Guidelines for prevention of stroke in patients with stroke and transient ischemic attack. *Stroke* 2014; 45: 2160–2236.

AHA/ASA guideline. Guidelines for the management of spontaneous intracerebral hemorrhage. *Stroke* 2015; 46: 2032–2060.

AHA/ASA guideline. Guidelines for the management of aneurysmal subarachnoid hemorrhage. *Stroke* 2012; 43: 1711–1737.

AHA/ASA guideline. Guidelines for the management of patients with unruptured intra-cranial aneurysms. *Stroke* 2015; 46: 2368–2400.

Bates B, Richards L, Ruff R, *et al.* Veterans Affairs/Department of Defense clinical practice guideline for the management of stroke rehabilitation. Version 3.0 2010. https://www.healthquality.va.gov/guidelines/Rehab/stroke (accessed June 2019).

AHA/ASA scientific statement. Management of stroke in neonates and children. *Stroke* 2019; 50: e51–e96.

AHA/ASA policy statement. Recommendations for the establishment of stroke systems of care: a 2019 update. *Stroke* 2019. doi:10.1161/STR.0000000000000173. [Epub ahead of print].

AHA scientific statement. Poststroke fatigue: emerging evidence and approaches to management. *Stroke* 2017; 48: e159–e170.

AHA scientific statement. Poststroke depression. *Stroke* 2017; 48: e30–e43.

AHA policy statement. Recommendations for the implementation of Telehealth in cardiovascular and stroke care. *Circulation* 2017; 135: e24–e44.

AHA/ASA scientific statement. Treatment and outcome of hemorrhagic transformation after intravenous alteplase in acute ischemic stroke. *Stroke* 2017; 48: e343–e361.

Index